Fitness for Kids and Teens

Thomas D. Fahey
Professor of Physical Education and Exercise Science
California State University, Chico
Chico, CA 95929

Although sports and physical activity generally have a positive effect on health, they are not without risk; medical consultation prior to the commencement of any exercise program is, therefore, advisable. The author and publisher of this book assume no responsibility or liability for injury resulting from any exercise program or other physical activity suggested in this book.

Library of Congress Cataloging in Publication Data
Fahey, Thomas D.
    Good-time fitness for kids.
    Includes index.
    1. Physical education for children.
    2. Physical fitness.
    3. Motor learning.
    I. Title
    GV443.F33   613.7'042   79-15882
    ISBN 0-88421-089-8

All rights reserved. This book is protected by copyright. No part of this book may be reproduced in any form or by any electronic or mechanical means, including photocopying, or utilized by any information storage and retrieval systems without permission in writing from the copyright owner, Dr. Thomas D. Fahey.

The publisher is not responsible (as a matter of product liability, negligence or otherwise) for any injury resulting from any material contained herein. This publication contains information relating to general principles of medical care that should not be construed as specific instructions for individual patients. Manufacturers' product information and package inserts should be reviewed for current information, including contraindications, dosages, and precautions.

Printed in United States of America.
Re-published by: International Sports Sciences Association
Santa Barbara, CA
Book Design: Alex Jacobs, alexjacobsdesign.com

Contents

Introduction 7

Young and Active 9

    Before Birth and Onward..10
    Creating Positive Experiences 11
    Fitness and Skills 16
    Instant Replay 29

Getting Off to a Fast Start: The Early Years 31

    The Child's Changing Body..32
    Motor Development During Infancy 35
    Motor Development During Childhood...39
    The Elementary School Physical Development Program 53
    Developing Basic Skills in Children 54
    Instant Replay 55

The Transition Years: Puberty and Adolescence 57

    The Body in Transition 58
    Motor Development During Adolescence 60
    Developing Endurance 62
    Developing Speed and Agility 69
    Developing Flexibility 72
    Developing Strength 76
    The School Physical Education Program 84
    Instant Replay 85

Competitive Athletics..87

How to Select the Right Sport **88**
Getting the Child Involved in Competitive Athletics **94**
Maximizing Your Child's Sports Experience **97**
Science and Athletics **100**
Girls and Athletics **104**
Bill of Rights for Young Athletes **105**
Instant Replay **105**

Athletic Injuries: Prevention and Treatment **107**

Preventing Injuries **107**
When to Call the Doctor **113**
Common Injuries and Disabilities in Children's Sports **114**
Instant Replay **121**

Developing an Active Lifestyle **123**

Sports, Exercise, and Health **123**
Developing Skills in Lifetime Sports **126**
Putting Sports in Perspective **134**
Instant Replay **134**

Index **136**

Introduction

Sports are an extremely important part of a child's life. If the athletic experience is positive, a child will develop a good self-image, a healthy body, and a large repertoire of sports that can be enjoyed for a lifetime. If, on the other hand, sports create a negative experience, a child may become bitter and guilt-ridden and may learn to hate physical activity. Mere participation in sports does not guarantee a positive athletic experience; just how beneficial it can be depends on guidance from parents, coaches, personal trainers, teachers, and other children, along with a positive attitude in the child. The purpose of this book is to present methods designed to acquaint any child with the joy of sports and to maximize his or her athletic potential.

Fitness for Kids and Teens is aimed at both the athlete and the non-athlete. For the athlete, it provides a birth-to-adulthood program designed to produce winning performance, and describes specific exercises that develop basic movement skills essential to sports. This comprehensive program includes information about training schedules, sports clubs, relationships with coaches, and enhancing emotional well-being through sports. For the non-athlete, the book describes a program that develops efficient movements, an appreciation for sports, and lifetime exercise habits which foster good health and enjoyment.

There are proven methods for helping to develop the athletic skill level in any child. Physical performance can be improved without causing emotional harm. The key, no matter what a child's level of ability, is to help him or her reach full athletic potential and share in a positive, enjoyable experience through sports.

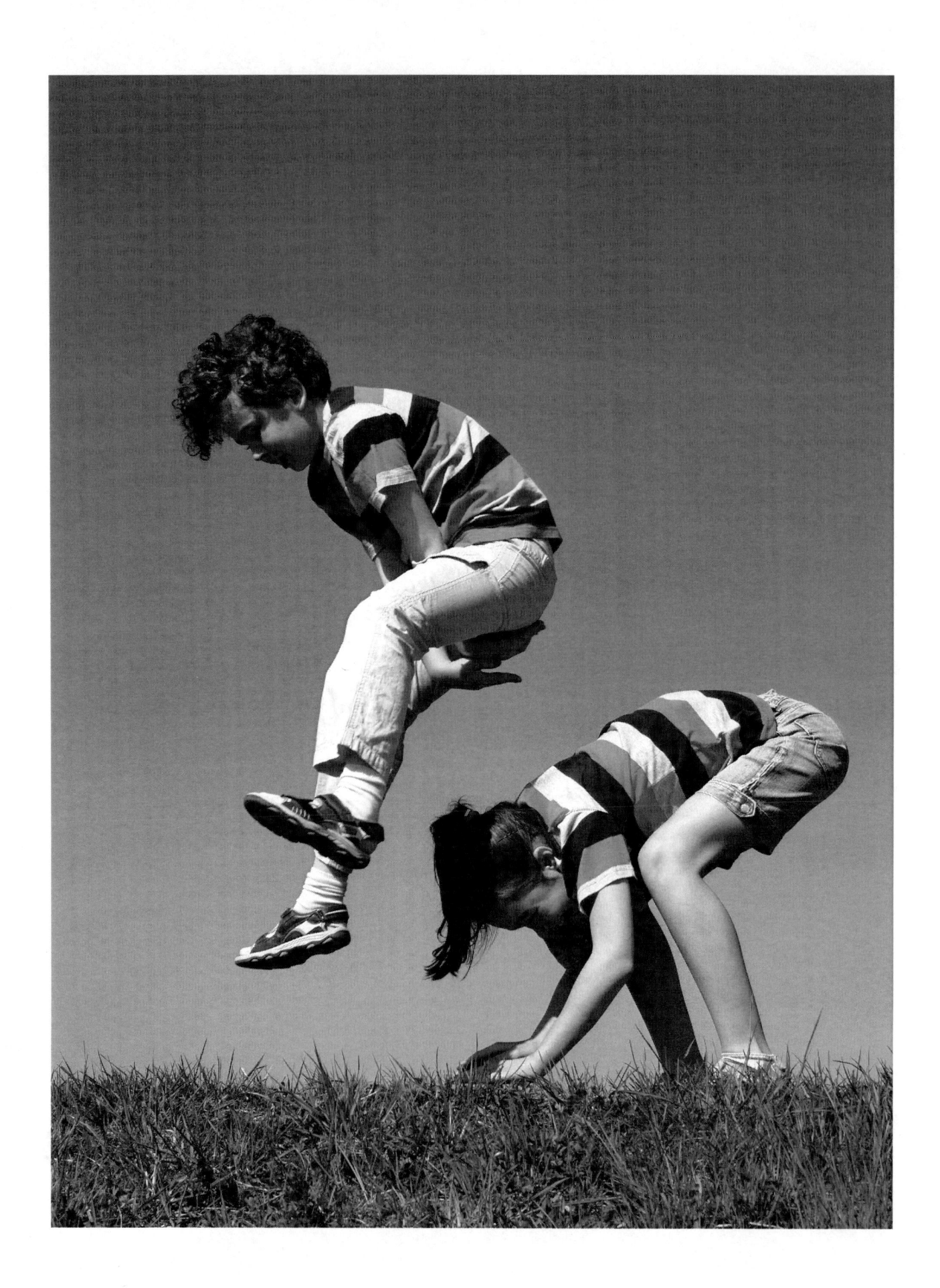

YOUNG & Active

Carol beamed as she ran into the house after her weekly soccer game. She was exhausted, but she had thoroughly enjoyed herself.

"Did you have a good time?" asked her father.

"I sure did! I made a great kick that almost went into the goal!"

"That's great, honey," exclaimed Carol's father. "Did your team win?"

"No—but one of these days we will. Every week we get better and better."

Carol is enjoying a positive experience in soccer and reaping all the benefits that sports have to offer—the classic benefits we heard about in old Pat O'Brien football movies: Sports build character, promote health, and increase vitality. Carol's positive experience will very likely encourage her to continue her participation in sports.

Sports and physical activity are vital to well-balanced development in boys and girls. A series of positive athletic experiences in childhood can lead to a lifetime of fitness, and will almost certainly create a lasting self-image of confidence and assuredness. Some children do not fare well under the rigors of competitive athletics and physical education programs. By getting caught up in the pressures of organized sports, they become physically or emotionally "burned out" at a very young age. Other children do not take part in competitive athletics at all; they shun physical activity for fear of not being able to perform up to the level of their peers. The negative effects on these "movement dropouts" can be life-long, since rejection of sports and physical activity in childhood will usually produce an adult who is overweight, sedentary, and less healthy than men and women who are athletically active.

Sports can be an extremely positive experience that will enhance the physical and emotional development of your child. But a positive experience doesn't happen by accident. As a parent, personal trainer, or coach, you have to provide the proper environment and emotional support for the necessary physical and psychological benefits to occur.

Throughout history, it was assumed that mere participation in sports produced positive effects. Plato said that a healthy mind and a healthy body went automatically hand in hand. Arthur Wellesley, the Duke of Wellington, attributed the English victory at Waterloo to sports participation at Eton (I guess they didn't have Little League parents in those days). Football coaches can talk for hours about the superior character they're developing in their players. Unfortunately, though, these romantic notions have not been supported by scientific evidence. Dr. Bruce Ogilvie, an internationally renowned sports psychologist, has stated that sports participation in certain programs is not necessarily beneficial to emotional development; in fact, the athletic experience can sometimes be harmful and psychologically traumatic. Programs that place unreasonable demands on children may cause permanent physical and emotional scars. As a parent, you can't let this happen.

Part of your responsibility to your child is to provide a healthy, positive atmosphere for physical activity and sports. You should encourage a variety of "movement experiences" and create a long-term program that will prepare your child for a lifetime of physical activity. The program should always be for the benefit of the child; it should be flexible enough to account for individual temperament, desires, and abilities. Temper the program with patience and understanding, and try constantly to increase your knowledge of exercise and its relationship to emotional and physical development. A long-term program will provide your child with the opportunity to get the full enjoyment and benefits of sport. And if the program takes into consideration your own growth as well as your child's, the sports experience will be a positive one for both of you.

Before Birth and Onward

Believe it or not, your preparation as a sporting parent begins even before the birth of your child. Recent scientific evidence suggests that a mother who exercises regularly during pregnancy will have a baby with a larger, more powerful heart. Be careful because excessive exercise—overtraining—can do the opposite. After the birth of the child, your job is to help your baby develop a varied perception of the world and allow him or her to develop full use of the body through exploration. As the baby becomes a toddler and then a school-age child, emphasize many kinds of physical activities. Be patient with your child's sometimes clumsy movements and slow progress; realize that the failures are just as important as the successes in the process of learning. To deny your child some failure is to stunt the learning process.

As a parent, teacher, coach, or personal trainer your job is to maximize the child's development. Every child develops at a different rate. Some show the skills and ability to become proficient athletes at an early age, while others are slower and may even appear athletically inept. Support the child! Sports and exercise are just as important for the less physically advanced child as they are for the budding superstar. Although it may be more fun to watch the star player on the local Little League team (especially if it's your child), that fat little kid with the butterfingers deserves as much attention because he or she needs a lot more help in developing skills.

As the child enters puberty, your job becomes even more difficult since this is a period of such drastic transition and change. You have to help the child deal with the feelings of insecurity engendered by a rapidly changing body. If used properly, sports and physical activity can be a vehicle for developing self-confidence and the independence required of an adult. You have to provide support, but be careful not to push too hard. You might make mistakes along the way, but if you honestly assess and act in the best interests of your child, the end result will be positive and successful.

During the high school years, help the child keep sports experience in its proper perspective. Sports during this period have profound social as well as physical effects. The parent must encourage the high-achieving athlete in the academic aspects of education so that the high school experience is well rounded. The parent must help the athlete take the long view. For example, an athlete who takes drugs to improve performance or ignores a serious injury to continue playing learns a bad lesson and could be adversely affected ten or fifteen years after graduation. Your advice can be tremendously helpful in assuring continued, long-term development.

The less physically skilled high school student needs parental guidance just as much. This person should be encouraged to continue the active lifestyle for its own sake. A lifetime of physical activity is a lot more important than a few years as a football hero. Encourage participation in sports for its intrinsic value. The lasting rewards of athletic involvement will benefit the high school superstar and the non-athlete alike.

Creating Positive Experiences

Movement and physical games come naturally to children. These experiences can and should develop a sense of self-worth, physical prowess, optimal health, and growth. They should also set the stage for a lifetime of physical activity. Although activity in the child is natural, you can encourage it by creating an ideal environment for movement and sports. For the baby, this involves providing opportunities for the manipulation of the surroundings (see Chapter 2 for a full discussion). For the child and teenager, it involves creating family and school atmospheres where sports participation are accepted lifestyles (see Chapters 2 to 4).

Winning — in the Personal Sense

You can make your child a winner! I'm not using the word winner in a Lombardian sense—that winning isn't everything, it's the only thing. A winner is a person who plays up to his or her potential. A winner can be a child who almost caught a ball. A winner can be the kid who lost a tennis match love-six, love-six, but hit the ball a little better than last time out. Self-improvement is the essence of winning. If you improve, you will be on the road of the winner.

What about winning and other people? If you continue to progress, you will eventually outperform other people. For most of us, there will always be someone who can move better, hit the ball harder, putt with more accuracy, or lift more weight. But through practice, you can and will improve. If you shun activity because you aren't performing as well as other people, the only person you're cheating is yourself. Unfortunately, many children do shun sports at a young age because they perceive themselves as failures. The child who is clumsy, or can't run very fast, or can't catch a ball as well as the other kids needs support and encouragement so that he or she can learn that improvement, slow as it may come, is success.

Stress small gains. Encourage the child to do one more pull-up, jump one-inch further, or hit one more ball over the net. Small, short-term goals are much easier to achieve than grand, unapproachable ones, such as making the Olympic team, playing in the Super Bowl, or becoming a professional bodybuilder or fitness model. Children may achieve these things if they make a series of small gains.

How important is winning in the traditional sense of conquering the opponent? Success in business depends on a person's ability to produce and perform better than others. Although idealists would have us believe that we can survive without being competitive, this idea is not consistent with reality. Adults are expected to pay bills on time, fulfill obligations to family, friends, and business associates, and conform to certain requirements of society. Of course, non-competitive person can reach high levels of performance in our society, but these are the exceptions rather than the rule. An adult must possess a certain amount of competitiveness to survive and get ahead. So, winning and excellence are important—but only under the proper circumstances. Children have to be taught how to win, lose, and overcome adversity

If we live in a competitive society, then why not expose children to the realities of winning and losing from the start? We don't for the same reason we don't send three-year-old babies to work: They are not physically, mentally, or emotionally prepared. Infancy, childhood, and adolescence are periods of development and learning. Early competition may result in cutting off the learning process prematurely. We know that the continued improvement of physical fitness, movement skills, perception, and personality depend on firm foundations. Skills learned during infancy serve as a foundation for skills learned during childhood, which in turn serve as the foundation for skills learned during adolescence. The ability to move gracefully and confidently as a teenager or adult originates in the experiences of earlier years. The more positive these experiences, the greater the likelihood of progressive improvement in skill and fitness.

De-emphasizing winning during childhood is not the same as abandoning excellence in movement skills. Many modern physical education experts place less emphasis on skill development and more on movement. Their philosophy is that learning motor skills is difficult and damages self-esteem. They substitute traditional motor skills, such as skipping rope, with skipping rope using an imaginary rope. Mastering sports skills—tennis forehands, the golf swing, throwing or catching a ball, or a carved ski turn—is challenging, frustrating, and difficult. Few important things are easy. Just as it takes work to master algebra, biology, or English, children have to work hard to master motor skills.

Winning is an important part of sports. When you win, you know you have performed well—or at least better than your opponent. However, the opponent you should concentrate on most is yourself. A child must have the chance to develop the tools for good performance. Introducing a progression of challenges to children in small steps prepares them for eventual competition with others. Early emphasis on competition and winning has the effect of stunting growth in a number of important skill and fitness areas: early competition causes premature specialization and distorts the meaning of winning. Children who learn to compete against themselves will become more confident, skillful teenagers and adults.

The vast majority of the nation's top youth coaches and athletic authorities agree that sports, during the earlier years, should be geared toward fun and the opportunity to have a large variety of experiences. There is nothing wrong with belonging to a children's football team, track club, or swim team, but the emphasis should be on developing fundamental movements and skills and fitness, not on intense competition or annihilating the opponent. Every child should get to play in all the games. Six- or seven-year-old children should not be barred from an athletic team because they are less skilled than the others. The bad experience of the rejected child far exceeds any good derived by the more skilled child. Except in sports where early participation is essential—figure skating, gymnastics, and swimming—children should avoid serious athletic competition before they are ten years old. Early athletic experiences are valu-

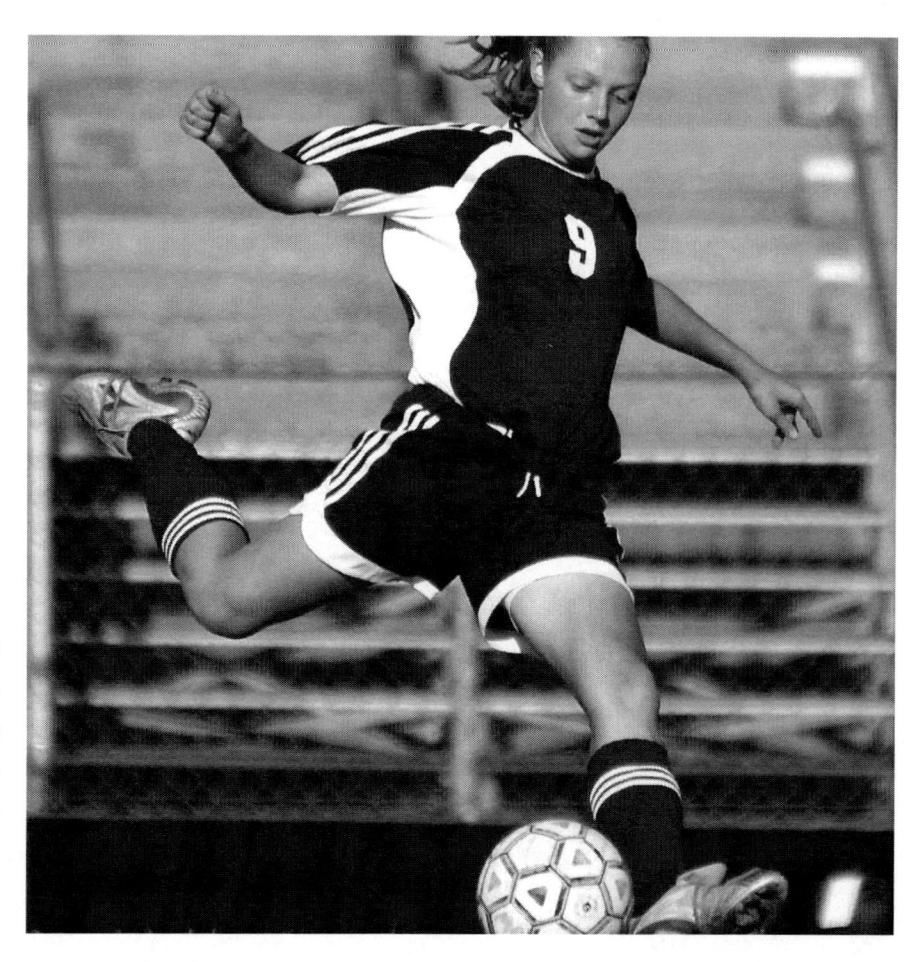

The ability to move gracefully as a teenager or adult is developed through athletic skills learned in childhood.

YOUNG AND ACTIVE | **13**

able for the child only if they provide fun and enhance continued development of fitness and skill. These experiences can provide an atmosphere for socialization, too. In the right environment, this socialization engenders self-confidence, tolerance of others, and sportsmanship. In the wrong environment, the childhood competitive experience creates a pubescent primadonna who can't cooperate with others and lacks the ability to improve.

An alternative to early competition is sports instruction. Children can take lessons in gymnastics, tennis, skiing, diving, horseback riding, dancing, and ice-skating—all in a non-competitive environment. Instruction is available in team sports through after-school programs, recreation departments, YMCA programs, scouting, and private clubs. Through these programs, the child can try out many different sports. A variety of experiences develops well-rounded skills and allows a more rational basis for sports specialization during the teenage years.

Competition is a vital part of sports, but your most important opponent is yourself.

The Family Environment

The best potential atmosphere for positive sports experiences is within the family. The parents must set a good example. If you, as a parent, exercise regularly and include sports as part of your lifestyle, you are creating a good environment for movement. Your children will grow up knowing that exercise and fitness are natural. Include your children in your physical activities. Scientists have discovered that even very young children are capable of exercise and have tremendous physical potential. Five- or six-year-old children can go on a two-mile run if they build up to it gradually. A three-year-old can begin skiing provided the sport is practiced in an atmosphere of fun and takes into consideration the physical comfort of the child.

Go on sports vacations. A camping vacation, for example, is a great way to expose your child to the rigors of hiking and instill an appreciation for the outdoors. Children relish these experiences even though their presence may sometimes be trying for the parents. A young child may need help carrying his equipment and may not be able to hike very far, but the experience of the trip will be unforgettable.

Taking an Interest

Positive sports experiences depend, in part, on parental support. You have to take an interest. Most coaches would rather deal with overbearing, meddling parents than with parents who don't care. They can channel the energy of the overly concerned parent into something beneficial for the team and the child. An unconcerned parent leaves the child high and dry. A child must get support from home to withstand the rigorous demands of competitive sports.

14 FITNESS FOR KIDS AND TEENS

Parental support must be tempered with tolerance and good sense. You have to let your child do it. You can't make your daughter shoot baskets better or your son run faster. You can create an atmosphere to assist improvement, but you can't force children to do something they are incapable of or don't want to do. A friend of mine, a former Olympic swimmer, told me that she would never forgive her father for ruining her childhood. Her father forced her to train long hours in the pool for the express purpose of winning an Olympic gold medal. He was never satisfied—she would swim her best time and her father would immediately plan for the next record-breaking performance. Nothing she could do seemed to satisfy him. If she didn't swim well at a meet, he would openly criticize her in front of her friends or criticize the coach. Although she made the Olympic team at a young age, she dropped out of swimming at the peak of her prime. She felt that her father was pushing her merely to satisfy his own ego.

Parental meddling can upset the non-athlete as well. I remember vividly the case of a thirteen-year-old boy whose parents brought him to my exercise physiology laboratory to stimulate his interest in sports. His father, who thought of himself as the pro-football coach type, told me that his son had no self-confidence, and that the other kids thought he was a sissy. The father said he would not stand for

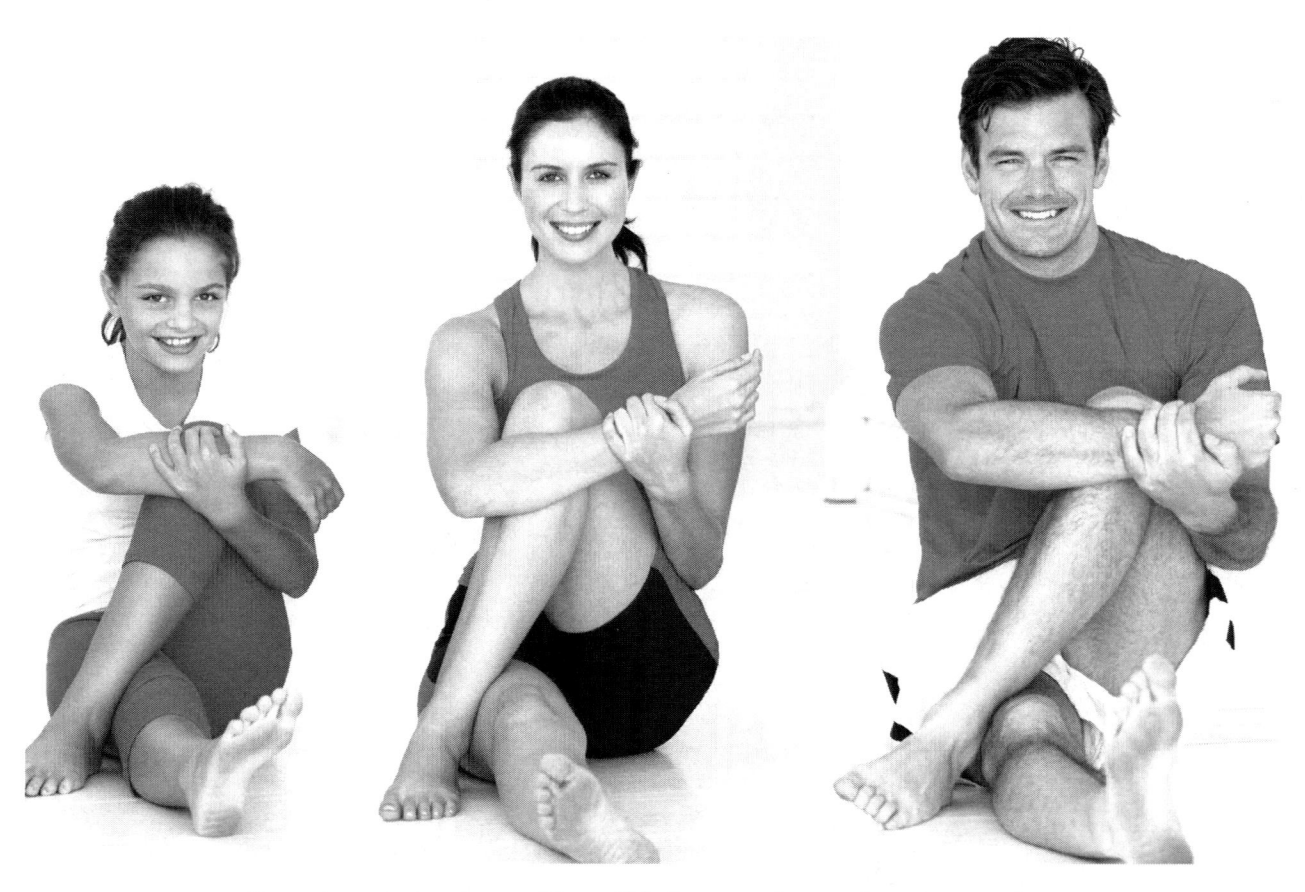

Parents can create positive athletic experiences by encouraging sports and participating in exercise with their children.

behavior in his son that was anything less than "100 percent he-man." He wanted to whip his son into shape and make a man out of him. In addition to the pressure the father exerted, the boy had a mother who would not let him think for himself—she even told me when the child was tired during his treadmill test. The parents refused to allow me to consult with the boy after his tests. They wanted to use the test results to further manipulate his behavior. It is little wonder that the child had no self-confidence and shied away from competition. He never had a chance to do things for himself. Although the boy's parents had good intentions, they did not create a good environment for a positive sports experience.

Not every child can become a successful athlete, regardless of the kind of sports environment provided. But most children can have positive athletic experiences if the atmosphere is right. Parents must open their minds to the benefits that can be gained by children in a sports program—even children of average ability. In addition to the physical benefits of exercise, sports can help with social and psychological development. Participation in sports is much more conducive to the maturing process than watching television all afternoon or joining a street gang. Gold medals and breakfast cereal endorsements aren't the only reasons to practice sports, although there isn't a week that goes by without some parent or coach asking me for a prediction of the physiological potential of an athlete: "If the kid doesn't have it, I want to know it now. I don't want to waste a lot of years training the child and find out it was all for nothing." Obviously, this attitude will not lay the best groundwork for positive experiences.

Fitness and Skills

Creating a positive sports experience involves systematically developing the physical, emotional, and skill abilities of your child. These abilities are specific—that is, distinct from one another. For example, if you work to develop endurance fitness, you will not necessarily develop strength fitness or motor skills. Your plan should be for a progression of improvement. In order to accurately determine the best program for the development of specific abilities and improvement progression, you need a basic understanding of the abilities. You should also understand the effect of growth and maturing on skills and physical fitness.

To maximize the sports experience, you must seek total, well-rounded development of the child. Emphasize activities appropriate for the child's age or stage of development. For instance, providing opportunities for play and movement exploration is much better for young children than channeling them into organized sports.

Endurance Fitness

Cardiovascular capacity is one the most important kinds of fitness you can help your child develop. Among adults, heart disease is the leading cause of death, and studies show that heart disease and obesity begin during childhood. Some of the leading risk factors include:

- High blood fats
- High blood pressure
- Obesity
- Smoking
- Lack of exercise

- High blood sugar and insulin resistance
- Male gender
- Family history
- Diabetes

Many studies show that the more endurance fitness a person has, the lower the risk of heart disease. Because adult habits form at a young age, it is easier to begin a fitness-oriented active lifestyle during the formative years than to adapt to it as a teenager or adult. In 1996, the US Surgeon General recommended that all Americans exercise moderately for 30 minutes a day. In 2002, the National Academies of Sciences increased this recommendation to 60-minutes of accumulated activity per day—if the goal is to maintain a healthy body weight. Health-related organizations such as the American Heart Association and American College of Sports Medicine recognize that participation in intense physical activities renders even more benefits.

The extent of endurance fitness reflects the amount of exercise children get and their natural ability—training and genetics. Studies of five-year-old children have shown them to have a remarkable capacity for endurance exercise. Yet, endurance exercise is not a natural part of the play of young children. While there is nothing wrong with endurance training in four- to eight-year-old children, some current practices, such as involving young children in serious competitive distance training in running and swimming, are irresponsible. It is difficult to comprehend that any five- or six year-old would run a marathon or even a 10-k run without being coerced into it by an overly zealous parent. Children can develop considerable age appropriate endurance by participating in a variety of sports and moderate endurance training activities.

Endurance training at a young age is perfectly okay if practiced in an atmosphere of fun and general family participation. Running clubs around the country get together regularly for fun runs and picnics in a non-competitive atmosphere. Exercising for fun gives a young child the chance to develop both physically and emotionally. When the time comes for rigorous training and competition, at about puberty, the child will be prepared. It makes no sense to have a fourteen-year-old boy or girl retire from sports because of early competition "burnout" during the elementary school years.

Endurance training has profound effects on a child's body. During their first five years, spontaneous play gradually increases the stamina of the growing child automatically. Varied sports participation during years five to ten further prepares the cardiovascular system, metabolism, and muscles for a lifetime of health and vigor. When heavy endurance training begins, the body's physiological systems start to become extremely specialized.

Endurance performance depends on the heart's ability to pump blood (cardiac output) and on well muscles' extract oxygen from the blood. Endurance training can, in some cases, increase the maximum cardiac output by an incredible 100 percent! Endurance training also improves the muscle's chemical systems by causing mitochondria, the energy centers of cells, to increase in both size and number. The result of endurance exercise, then, is to improve both oxygen transport and oxygen utilization. Both of these factors improve ability to perform more exercise for a longer period of time.

Endurance fitness is important for children regardless of whether or not they ever seriously enter competitions. Endurance exercise is critical to a healthy body that is free from the risk of heart disease, but it is also important for maintaining enough energy to stay alert for daily activities. Endurance exercise is also a primary method of controlling body fat, which is a serious problem among today's children. Endurance fitness is necessary so your child has the stamina to participate in a well-rounded, physically active lifestyle. Endurance fitness should be of primary concern throughout childhood development.

Probably the best measure of the fitness of the cardiovascular system is the maximal oxygen consumption test (called $\dot{V}O_2$ max by scientists). $\dot{V}O_2$ max, measured in the sports medicine laboratory, collects respiratory gases expired by a test subject as he or she runs on a treadmill or rides a stationary bicycle. The person being tested looks like an astronaut who has just returned from Venus: exotic headgear supports a valve and tube for breathing, electrodes and wires are attached to the chest, and a blood pressure cuff is wrapped around the arm. To make things worse, the nose is plugged so the subject can only breathe through the mouth. The person is then expected to run to exhaustion as laboratory assistants watch little television screens that display the computer's findings on the measurements taken during the test!

The $\dot{V}O_2$ max determines a person's capacity for endurance exercise. Olympic-caliber athletes who compete in distance running and swimming and cross-country skiing have maximal oxygen consumption capacities that far exceed those of the average person. Top athletes can typically consume from 75 to almost 90 milliliters of oxygen per kilogram of body weight each minute, while the average person can take in only about 35 to 50 milliliters. Top endurance athletes are born with much of this

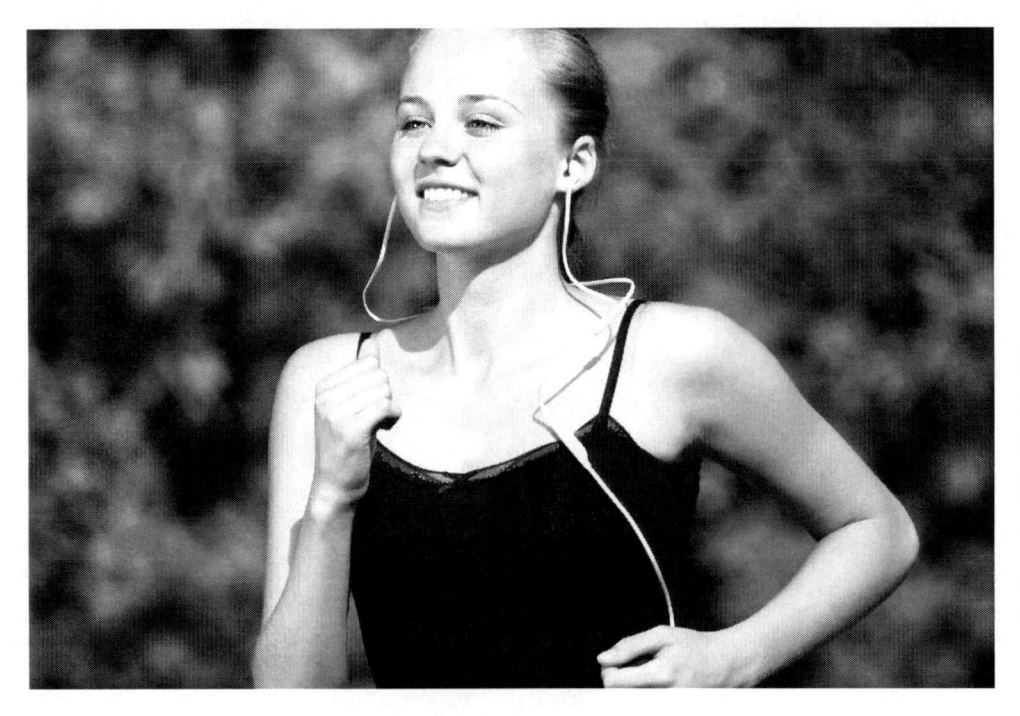

Endurance exercise is essential for maintaining a healthy body and for promoting stamina and a high energy level.

capacity. Dr. Per-Olaf Åstrand, a world-famous Swedish exercise physiologist, estimates that to become a world-class endurance athlete, a male must possess a minimum $\dot{V}O_2$ max of about 65 milliliters of oxygen per kilogram of body weight—before active training begins. For females, a prospective world-class athlete must possess at least 55 milliliters. All world-class distance runners belong to the high $\dot{V}O_2$ max club. Endurance athletes must combine natural ability with years of exhaustive and arduous training—then they may have a chance to achieve the top.

That may sound like a pretty bleak picture to those of us with a lower capacity. Yet anyone, at any age, can greatly improve oxygen consumption capacity by regular and systematic endurance exercise. One of the major functions of my laboratory is to measure oxygen consumption capacity and help people design exercise and training programs to help them improve. I have found this invaluable for helping children choose the sports for which they're best suited, and for making them aware of their current fitness level.

I do not believe treadmill tests are particularly valuable for children younger than eight years. Before this age, children lack the maturity—or perhaps the stupidity—to run to exhaustion on a treadmill. I learned this lesson the hard way. During my first year as an exercise physiologist, I observed an age-group track meet where I saw a six-year-old boy, with no competitive experience, run a mile in six minutes and 53 seconds. Jimmy seemed to revel in the cheers from the stands and his parents adoration. I went up to his mother after the race and asked if I could test the boy in my laboratory. I didn't know much about the exercise capacity of children then, and thought this would be the perfect opportunity to learn.

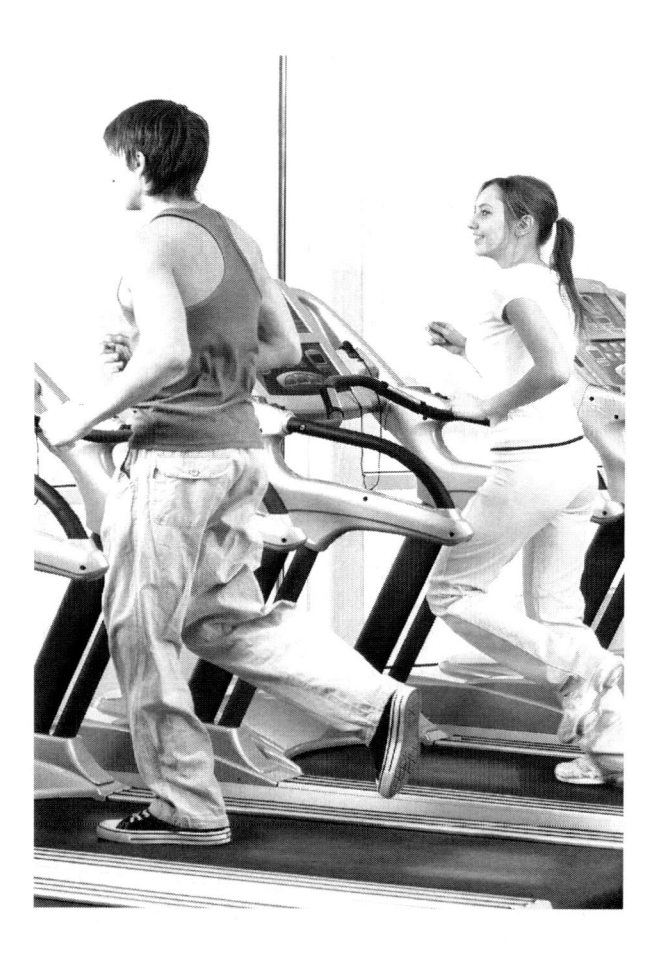

Jimmy's father practically had to drag him into the lab. To make matters worse, Jimmy was scared to death of my laboratory assistant, Lahsen Akka, a 275-pound Olympian from Morocco who was the African record holder in the shot-put and discus. The little boy's nose was so small we had to tape it closed because we couldn't use the standard nose clip. We prepared him for the test, but he really didn't understand what was happening to him. The first few minutes on the treadmill went pretty well. Then Lahsen turned up the speed of the treadmill, and the boy started to cry (which was pretty tough because he had a tube in his mouth). A little while later it was time to increase the speed again. Jimmy could see Lahsen going for the speed button and became panic stricken. At that point, Lahsen and I looked at each other and decided to stop the test.

The experience of the treadmill in the lab was considerably different from the enjoyable atmosphere of the track meet. The little boy could not understand why running, which was so much fun for him on the track, was now connected to some bizarre torture. It's better to wait until a child becomes seriously specialized in competitive endurance sports before getting a treadmill evaluation.

A treadmill test is valuable for any child who becomes serious about competitive endurance athletics. The best place for a young athlete to get a treadmill test at a sports sciences laboratory that specializes in physical performance analysis. Such labs exist in the physical education departments of universities across the country. Several private sports medicine clinics also provide this service. Although most hospitals perform the treadmill test, they are seldom equipped to provide knowledgeable advice about endurance training. Hospital treadmill tests are usually conducted to diagnose heart diseases, and few physicians have enough knowledge of athletics or exercise training methods to justify the expense of a hospital treadmill test for a healthy child.

The United States Olympic Committee has Olympic development training centers at Colorado Springs, Colorado; San Diego, California; and Lake Placid, New York. These centers were established specifically to aid elite and promising young athletes with the the potential to be champions, and offer them the opportunity to receive performance analysis from sports medicine experts. Your child can find out about these programs by contacting one of these centers. The governing bodies of various Olympic sports extend invitations to young athletes to attend the centers who have the potential of making the Olympic teams someday.

It is possible to estimate the results a child can obtain on a treadmill with the 1.5-mile run test (described in Chapter 3). When you know the child's endurance capacity, you can develop a program that will systematically increase cardiovascular capacity. In Chapter 3, there are simple-to-use charts that will aid you in increasing the endurance of any child safely and quickly.

Muscle Strength, Speed, and Power

Muscle fitness plays an extremely important part in athletic performance. It is very difficult to develop this type of fitness significantly until puberty, a time characterized by rapid growth and sexual maturing in boys and girls. During childhood, or up to about ten years of age for girls and about eleven or twelve for boys, it's best to emphasize exercise and sports that require the use of the whole body. Activity periods are better spent developing various movement skills rather than trying to systematically develop muscle strength through activities such as weight training. However, after puberty has begun, try to improve muscle fitness systematically. After puberty, bone, muscle, and nerves are mature enough and hormone function optimal for the development of speed and strength.

(There are programs to develop muscle strength and speed in Chapter 3.)

A certain amount of exercise is necessary for normal muscle growth. However, the extent of the development of a muscle's strength, power, and speed depends directly on the kind and amount of exercise the muscle is subjected to. Although performance depends, to a large extent, on inherited abilities, the training and experience a child receives throughout growth is a critical factor. The physical activities of childhood, such as climbing, skipping, running, and jumping, are very important for building a body that is capable of vigorous, specialized muscle training during the teenage years.

Muscle fitness does not mean merely increasing muscle size. Strength, power, and speed depend on a smooth coordination between the nervous system and the muscles. In fact, muscles are sometimes called the slaves of the nervous system. Nerves use different muscle fibers selectively as part of a process called recruitment. When you perform fast movements, your nervous system calls upon (recruits) muscle fibers designed for fast contraction. More muscle fibers are recruited to pick up a heavy object than a light one. Recruitment is the body's way of performing a movement efficiently. The efficiency of a person's recruitment is probably the most important single factor in separating the fast runner from the slow runner, the strong athlete from the weak athlete, and the skilled person from the unskilled person.

Muscle fibers are the basic components of a muscle. Nerves recruit muscle fibers depending upon the desired movements. The muscle fibers you use to run fast are different from the ones you use to jog. Fine manipulative tasks, such as threading a needle, demand the recruitment of different muscle fibers more than tasks like lifting a heavy weight. The nervous system has the ability to selectively recruit the muscle fibers that are best suited for either explosive movements or movements requiring endurance.

Fibers of skeletal muscles are divided into two major groups: fast twitch and slow twitch. Fast-twitch muscle fibers are further divided into two sub-categories, Type IIa and Type IIx. Slow-twitch muscle fibers are used when power and strength are required. Since most people have an equal distribution of fast- and slow-twitch muscle fibers, the average person has a pretty good ability to improve strength, speed, and endurance. Certain types of athletes have a predominance of one type of fiber over another. Top marathon runners, for example, have many more slow-twitch muscle fibers than fast-twitch fibers. Likewise, athletes who require explosive strength, such as sprinters, have a predominance of fast-twitch fibers.

Young people usually self-select the most appropriate activities for their predominant fiber and body type. A fast powerful child will naturally chose activities, such as sprinting, football or softball because those sports bring the most success. Slower, less powerful children may chose endurance activities because they are better suited to their capacity. Your job is to help channel children into activities where they will find enjoyment and success.

Hormones also play a prominent role in the development of muscle fitness. Androgen hormones, such as testosterone serve as the primary factor involved in the large increase

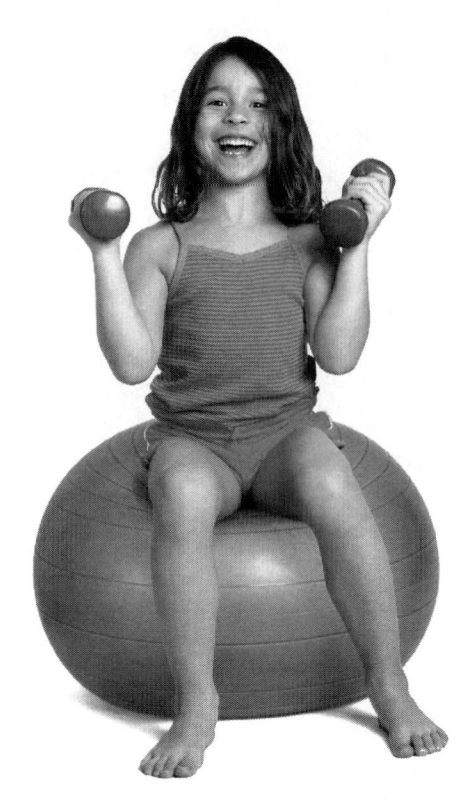

The physical activities of childhood can increase the body's capability for vigorous training in later life.

in muscle mass in boys during puberty. Testosterone is over ten times more abundant in sexually mature teenage boys than in girls. This hormone accounts for the large differences in strength, speed, and power that exist between men and women. These differences begin to manifest themselves during puberty, when there is an increased secretion of testosterone in boys. Girls, who do not secrete large amounts of testosterone, do not experience the large increases in muscle mass or strength during puberty.

Weight training will increase strength in girls, but will usually not increase muscle bulk—unless they have high levels of testosterone. Girls do experience a certain amount of hormone-related muscle changes (from small amounts of male hormones and other hormones that affect growth) through strength training exercises, but most of the improvement in performance is probably due to an increased efficiency and communication between nerves and muscle in the muscle recruitment patterns.

Building Strong Bones: Start When You're Young

Most people think of bones as big, solid structures—like rock walls—that give your body form and strength. Bone is a surprisingly active tissue. Bone cells continuously dissolve old bone and replace it with new bone so that your skeleton stays fresh and strong. During growth, you build more bone than you break down. This causes you to get taller and bigger and develop stronger bones.

Bones grow nearly continuously until you reach your late teens or early 20s. Bone density reaches a peak during your early to late 20s. After that, bone density decreases slowly and continuously as long as you live. With aging, the best you can hope for is to slow the rate of bone loss.

Bone researchers stress the importance of "banking bone" while you are young—building up as much bone as possible between ages 8 to 30. Bone banking will buffer the effects of gradual bone loss during the rest of your life. If you're older than 25 or 30 years, you can't do much about your peak bone density. But, you can prevent further bone loss—at least to an extent.

Weight training—and weight-bearing exercise in general—are the best ways to build and bank bone. Scientists have discovered important facts about exercise and weight training that you should consider when designing your program.

• Free weight exercises place more stress on the skeleton, so they are better than machine exercises for building bone. For example, weight machine leg presses build the spinal bones very well but don't stress the hips. Squats and lunges work better than leg presses because they force all the major bones in your lower skeleton to take more stress.

• Walking and running will build more bone density than cycling or similar non-weight bearing exercises (e.g., supine bicycle). Swimmers actually have lower bone density than normal because the body doesn't weigh very much in the water. No aerobic exercise will build bone the way weight training does. Lift weights 2 to 3 days weekly for optimal bone health.

• Bone responds best to high-tension exercises. Children shouldn't just go through the motions when they train—they must exercise hard. Bone responds to the stress of exercise and the pull of muscle on bone surfaces. Work hard for strong bones.

• The rate of applying stress to bone is more important than the absolute stress. Loading should be greater than everyday activities. Most children—particularly girls—should include box jumping in their bone preservation program. Box jumping (jumping from a 2 foot high box to the ground, then jumping up again) should be included in every child's physical education program. This type of exercise builds bone much better than jumping in place or jumping rope.

• Bones only respond to exercise when they have been stressed. If you stress spinal bones, you can't assume that you're also stimulating hipbones. Standing weight training exercises—such as squats, lunges, step-ups, and dead lifts—are best for loading the skeleton. Some researchers suggest that children wear weighted vests during exercise so that they can better load the bones of the spine, hip, and legs.

• If you stop loading your bones (i.e., stop exercising) you will lose any gains you made during your weight training program. You don't have to do many exercises to promote bone health. Even if you do only a few exercises a week, the extra bone load will protect them.

• Exercise can only build bone so much. Almost all growing children (grades 6 to 12) can increase bone density by doing weight bearing exercise, plyometrics (box jumping). These exercises should be required for all school children. Once they hit their 20's and 30's, they should work hard to maintain peak bone density for as long as possible. Bone deteriorates after about age 35, with a large decrease in bone density occurring during the first few years of menopause. Bone deteriorations may be prevented—at least in some women—through hormone replacement therapy, diets high in calcium, and high stress exercise.

• Young bone responds to exercise better than old bone does. So, it's vital that you begin your bone-building program as early as possible. The best time to start your program is in elementary school. Training in your 20s and 30s is good but not as good as beginning early. However, even women in their 70s and 80s can benefit from exercise and skeletal loading—provided it's done safely and under supervision.

- Do not expect changes overnight. Bone scans of women on weight training programs show that increases in bone density take about nine months.

- Strong muscles build strong bones. Build muscles through a combination of high tension weight training exercises and jumping.

Flexibility

A rule of medicine and physiology that's important for people to remember throughout life is that if you don't use it, you'll lose it. Babies are extremely flexible—it seems they can almost tie themselves in a knot. Because of muscular movements that utilize only restricted ranges of motion, flexibility in many joints is greatly diminished in many children by the time they become teenagers.

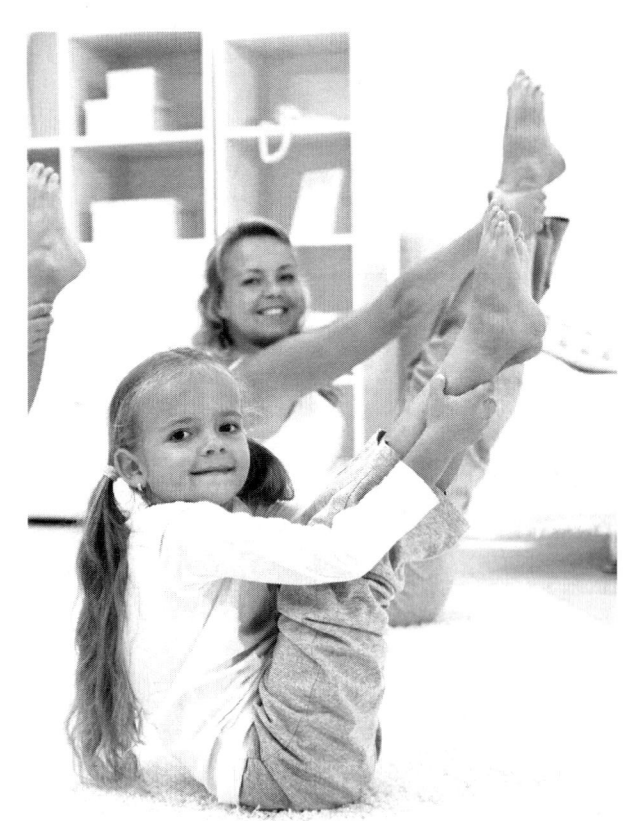

This gradual loss of flexibility has a price as the child gets older—an increased risk of athletic injuries, and the appearance of pain in areas such as the back and neck that can become chronic.

Boys generally lose flexibility much faster than girls. This probably results from patterns of play and physical activity rather than any pre-existing sex difference. Boys have traditionally participated in activities requiring speed and strength, such as football and baseball. These sports don't require body parts to move through large ranges of motion, so they gradually lose flexibility. Girls, on the other hand, often participate in gymnastics and dance, activities that require a great deal of flexibility. Children should practice flexibility exercises even before they enter school. Initially, they should develop flexibility by doing whole body movements (playing on bars, ropes, and ladders). After age five, children can begin formal flexibility exercises. If these are fun for them, children will keep their interest in maintaining flexibility. If children maintain the flexibility they had as babies, they won't have to work as hard as teenagers and adults to get it back.

Introducing flexibility exercises at an early age will help children maintain flexibility as they age.

Perceptual-Motor Skills

Last winter, while skiing at Mammoth Mountain in California, I watched a junior ski team working on the downhill, one of the most dangerous and difficult events in sports. I looked up at a steep ridge and saw a young racer in a tuck position zooming down the course—she must have been going faster than 75 miles per hour. She hit a particularly nasty rut and was thrown momentarily off balance. She ascended into the air, and somehow managed to land on both skis and finish her practice run. I was absolutely amazed-the course was solid ice, yet this thirteen-year-old girl was doing everything in her power to go as fast as she could. I had hesitated skiing down the same hill using dozens of turns; she went practically straight down. When the little girl finished her run, she took off her helmet and skis, walked over to her mother, and asked, "Can I play with my friends now?" Skiing was second nature to the young girl. Her skills were developed to such a point that she lacked the fear that adults who take up skiing at a later age usually have.

If you fail to learn certain motor skills at critical stages of development, you may never reach your full potential in a sport. A child progresses from one point to another in learning movement skills because each skill serves as a foundation for the next. To maximize the learning of complex motor skills, such as catching a football while avoiding a tackle or executing a spin on ice skates, the child must first master a series of more fundamental skills. Once children build a repertoire of movement patterns, they can develop more specific skills.

Children learn best by trial and error. The trick is to put children in situations where trial-and-error learning is constructive. This process should begin as soon as the baby arrives. From the very beginning, babies learn about their relationship with the world through experimentation. If the baby is given the opportunity to experience the world in unique ways, the learning that occurs will serve as the basis for the learning of more complex tasks later on.

What is the nature of trial-and-error learning? Trial-and-error learning is similar to the geographical learning that occurs when a person drives a car. Ask yourself this question, "Who learns the road better—the driver of the car or the passenger?" Both driver and passenger are going to the same place. The driver, though, is actively learning the geography by watching the road and determining which is the correct route and which is the incorrect. The passenger, on the other hand, is lead along the correct road without playing an active role in determining the correct path. Likewise, children cannot be shown how to do a particular movement and then learn it by osmosis. They must approach and master the task by themselves. Through trial and error and experience, children develops a catalog of movement skills that are later integrated into proficient sports techniques.

The ability to learn complex movements depends on a child's previous movement experiences. Every complex movement, such as hitting forehand in tennis, dribbling a basketball, hitting a softball, or doing somersault, incorporates a number of fundamental movement abilities. Hitting a forehand, for example, requires such basic movement and perception skills as tracking the ball visually, coordinating the hand and the eye, feeling the location of various body parts (kinesthesis), and maintaining balance while shifting body weight. To hit a forehand, these skills, and some other basic movement patterns, must be coordinated. If a child lacks experience in any of the fundamental movements, the more complex skill—forehand—will be more difficult to learn.

Basic skills are specific—this means that learning one basic movement skill does not result in the learning of another. For example, if a child works on balance skills, he or she won't be doing anything to develop hand/eye coordination. Children must develop a varied repertoire of specific basic movement patterns if they hope to develop more complex movement skills of sports. The more varied a child's fundamental movement experiences, the easier will be the mastery of more complex tasks. Exposure to basic movement patterns doesn't happen by accident, though. In order to maximize children's potential for skilled complex movement later in life, you must systematically expose them to a variety of movement experiences.

What are the specific movement skills that are important for complex sports techniques? Basic skills are grouped as perceptual and motor. Perceptual skills involve interpreting the sensory input from the outside world, and determine the body's ability to perceive its relationship to the environment. For example, if a ball is thrown at a child, the child must first recognize that the action has occurred; then he must be able to track the ball visually and to feel where his body parts are when he moves to catch the ball. Motor skills involve the body's reacting to this sensory information. To go back to the thrown ball, motor skills are the actual movements involved in catching the ball. Naturally, perceptual and motor skills are interdependent. Skilled movements require an integration of sensory and motor skills.

Kinesthesis, an extremely important perceptual skill, involves the recognition of the body's position in space. For example, if you stretch your arm out to one side, you can tell without looking and without moving where your fingers are and what position they're in, even though they are not touching anything. This perceptual skill can be developed from Day One, simply by changing the position in which you hold your baby. Climbing, walking on stairs and ladders, hanging on monkey bars, and moving in water provide young children with the opportunities to develop a feeling of the body's position in space.

Related to kinesthesis are laterality and directionality. Laterality is the ability to distinguish between the right and the left sides of the body. Directionality is the ability to distinguish the possible directions a movement may take. Even professional athletes have deficiencies in the basic skills of laterality and directionality. For example, some pro-tennis players move to one side better than to the other. Many top skiers can turn better to one side than the other.

Body image is an important early skill that children must learn in order to effectively understand their relationship with the environment. This skill involves developing an intuitive knowledge of body parts and what they are capable of doing.

Vision is an extremely important factor in movement. Visual ability involves a lot more than the capacity to read the big "E" on the eye chart. Effective vision involves the child's ability to use the ocular system (the eyes and the brain) dynamically. Visual tracking, the ability to watch a moving object, is extremely important for complex sports skills like catching a football or hitting a tennis ball. Visual tracking is a basic perceptual skill that can only be effectively developed if the child is given visual tracking experience. For example, babies can learn to focus on objects and follow their movements earlier if they are exposed to appropriate stimuli, such as moving mobiles. Early visual tracking experience is the ideal basis for more complex visual skills that may ultimately culminate in the ability to shag fly balls in Yankee Stadium, or catch the big one in the Super Bowl. Many ophthalmologists and optometrists can help determine your child's ability to use his ocular system effectively for sports. Eyesight is a critical sense for success in sports. Sensory-motor exercises will be more valuable if your child's visual system is operating at the optimal level.

Effective vision also requires visual-motor control—that is, the integration of vision with movement skills. Two of the most important components of visual-motor control are hand/eye coordination and foot/eye coordination, in which the eyes and the hands or feet work together to perform a task. Hand/eye and foot/eye coordination are task specific—proficiency in one does not result in proficiency in the other. Many children in the United States have excellent hand/eye coordination but poor foot/eye coordination. The reverse is true of most European children because of the different emphases in sports and movement experiences within their culture. Until recently, soccer, a sport requiring mostly foot movements, was more popular in Europe than in the United States. Most sports popular in this country, such as football, baseball, and basketball, are upper body oriented. In the past, most Americans began their soccer playing in high school or college, and so they lacked the childhood movement experiences that could have resulted in top performance in the ranks of profes-

Balance: a complex group of skills

sional soccer. Now, soccer is the fastest growing youth sport in the country, and early experiences are increasing. In future years, U.S. team players will be better represented in professional soccer, and the United States may even have a shot at the World Cup, the symbol of world soccer excellence.

Balance, the ability to maintain a posture against the forces of gravity, is another very complicated skill, or, more precisely, group of skills. Balance skills can be roughly grouped into static and dynamic categories. Static balance is required to remain still against gravity, while dynamic balance is the ability to control your body against gravity when you're moving. An example of static balance is standing in an upright position or standing on one foot. When you ski or run, dynamic balance is required in order to remain upright. Give children plenty of opportunities to balance themselves if you want to improve static and dynamic balance skills. Balance is often neglected because parents are fearful. Most parents become extremely apprehensive when they see a child who can't walk try to climb a ladder or try to make it down a flight of stairs. But it's important that children have these opportunities. You can keep an eye on an adventuresome child without preventing his or her explorations. A good amount of freedom of movement is required for a child to develop movement skills and the ability to react effectively to unique movement opportunities. Children who have a lot of movement experience move better than kids who don't.

Coordination is the end result of a child's ability to translate perception stimuli into effective movements. Coordinated movements are efficient and almost reflex in nature. You should remember that coordination is not a single entity, but a sum total of perceptual and motor skills. It is surprising how even professional coaches fail to understand this simple principle. Football coaches often talk about the importance of developing quick reaction time in their players. But reaction time is only one component of a sports movement; just as important is movement time. Complex sports

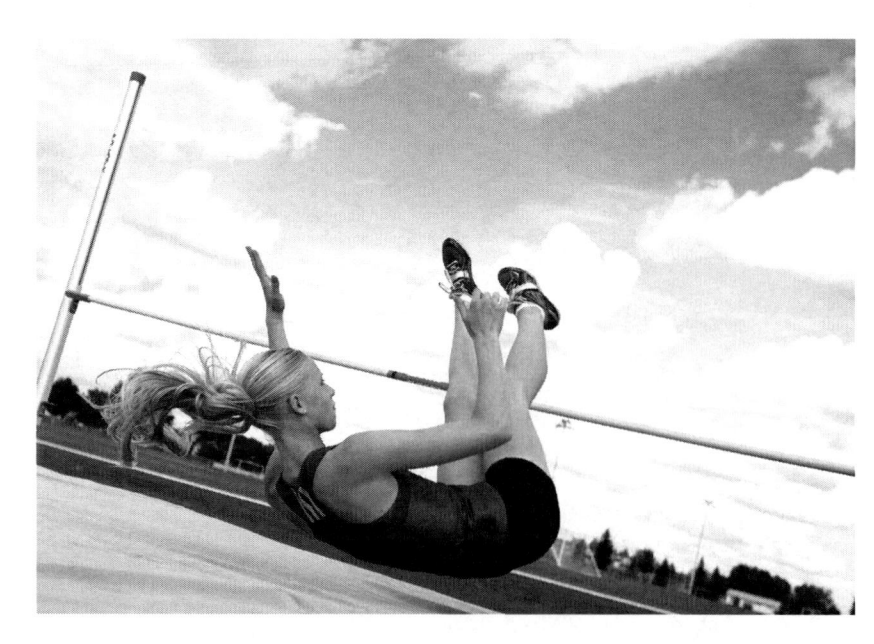

Highly developed sports techniques, such as the high jump, can only be developed through systematic practice of many different movement skills.

28 FITNESS FOR KIDS AND TEENS

techniques require effective reaction time (perceptual) and movement time (motor) alike. Techniques involving much coordination call for a good repertoire of basic movement skills and systematic practice of the actual skill. For example, proficiency at tennis requires good basic movement skills (the ability to start and stop, change directions rapidly, watch the ball, etc.) as well as practice on specific skills like forehands, backhands, serves, and volleys. If a person had a variety of movement experiences as a child, then coordinated sports techniques will result. The experienced person will be able to exhibit these coordinated movements in a variety of circumstances.

Tying It All Together

Skilled sports techniques depend upon the ability to effectively integrate physical fitness (endurance, strength, speed, power, and flexibility), perceptual abilities (eyesight, ocular tracking, kinesthetic perception), and motor abilities (movement time, hand/eye coordination, balance). All of these components are specific, and time must be spent on each factor throughout the period of growth and development. The best way to give your child an effective movement education is to provide the maximum opportunities for a variety of movement experiences.

Instant Replay

- Sports participation is not automatically a positive experience for the child. Care must be taken to provide the maximum opportunities for the development of skill and fitness. Early emphasis on competition may cause some children to drop out of sports prematurely.
- Children should be exposed to a variety of movement experiences from the first day of life on.
- Competition is important, but only after the child has had the opportunity to develop basic movement skills and self-confidence. Self-improvement is the most meaningful competition—it will ultimately result in the ability to defeat the opponent.
- Family participation in fitness activities develops positive attitudes about sports.
- Endurance fitness is important for the prevention of heart disease. This type of exercise develops the body's cardiovascular and chemical systems. The maximal oxygen consumption test measured on a treadmill or stationary bicycle is the best way to measure endurance fitness. Children should exercise at least 60-minutes a day.
- Muscle strength, speed, and power are specific to exercise training. Muscle fitness reflects the type of exercise the body is subjected to.
- Childhood exercise patterns set the stage for healthy bones throughout life. All elementary school children should practice exercises that build bone mass.
- Flexibility should be consistently and systematically maintained throughout life. "If you don't use it, you'll lose it."
- Basic movement patterns serve as the foundation for more complex movement skills. Movement experiences should be introduced according to the child's level of development.

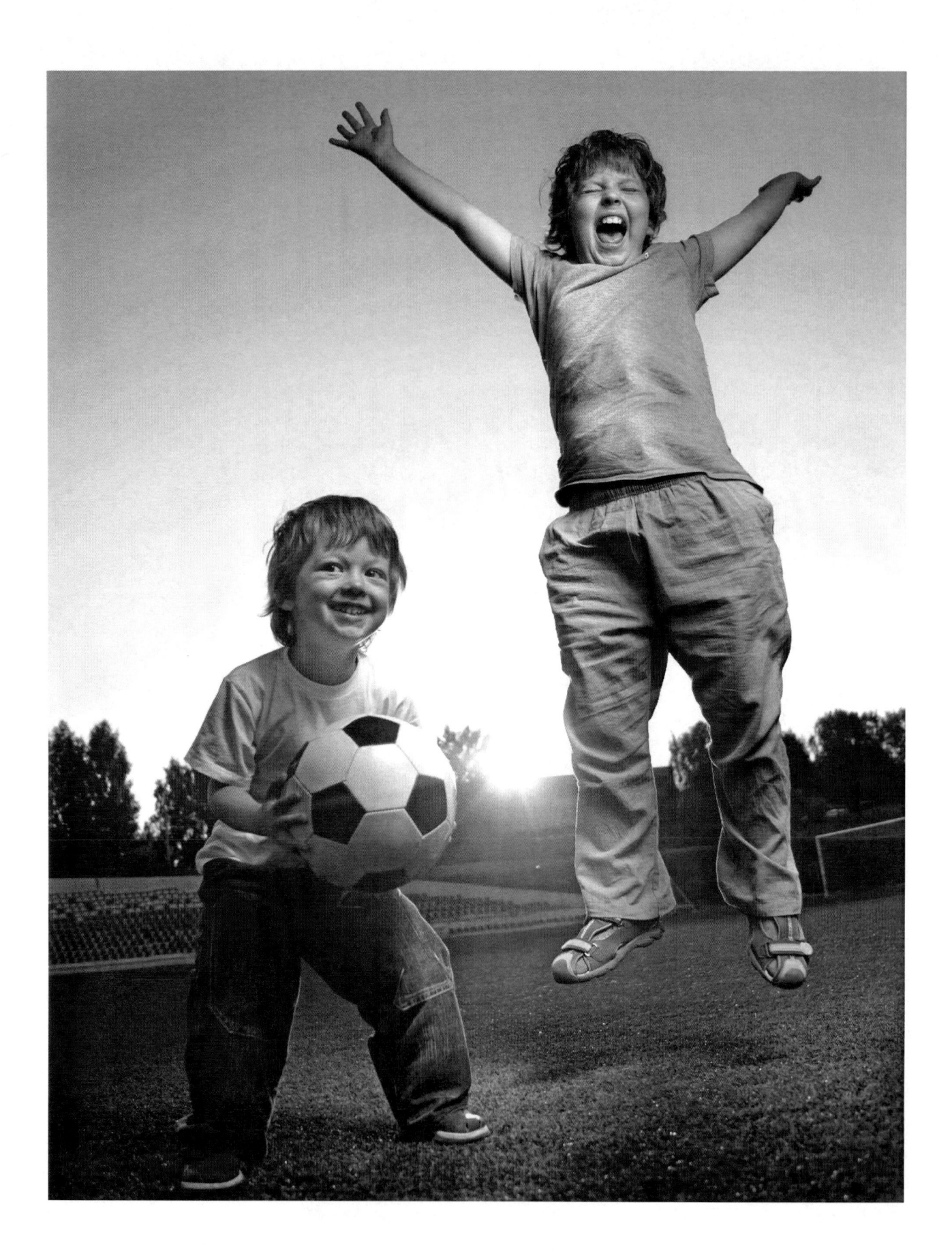

Getting Off to a Fast START

THE EARLY YEARS

"Why can't Jill be more like Teddy? Teddy is such a good boy—he just stays in his playpen and doesn't bother anyone. Now Jill, she's another story. She's always into everything. Turn your back on her for a minute and she starts climbing on the furniture. I'm afraid she's going to break her neck. Jill's behavior is her mother's fault. She lets her have too much freedom. Teddy's mother has the right idea—put him in the playpen so she can keep an eye on him."

Jill and Teddy were cousins who were raised under two different philosophies. Jill's parents believed that a variety of experiences were essential to both intellectual and motor development. They took precautions to childproof the house—they put safety locks on cabinets and moved delicate objects away from reach—but they only restricted her movements when they truly interfered with the rights of others. Jill's parents believed that even though they would be somewhat inconvenienced at times by giving Jill more freedom of movement, they would be giving their daughter the opportunity to fully develop her potential for efficient movement. Jill's parents were not permissive—they taught their daughter that some types of behavior were inappropriate.

Teddy, on the other hand, was restricted more than necessary. He was put into a playpen so he would be less trouble. Teddy was deprived of the opportunity for a variety of movement experiences. He was considered by some members of the family to be the model child. He was not as curious as Jill partly because his environment limited his curiosity. To casual outside observers, Teddy was viewed as cooperative and easy to get along with, but his development was impeded.

Which philosophy is most beneficial to the child's development? Most motor-development specialists agree with the philosophy of Jill's parents: to let the child have as much freedom of movement and as much stimulation as possible. As a result, the child will have the best opportunity to develop basic movement skills. These skills are not developed by accident, but by systematic exposure to new situations.

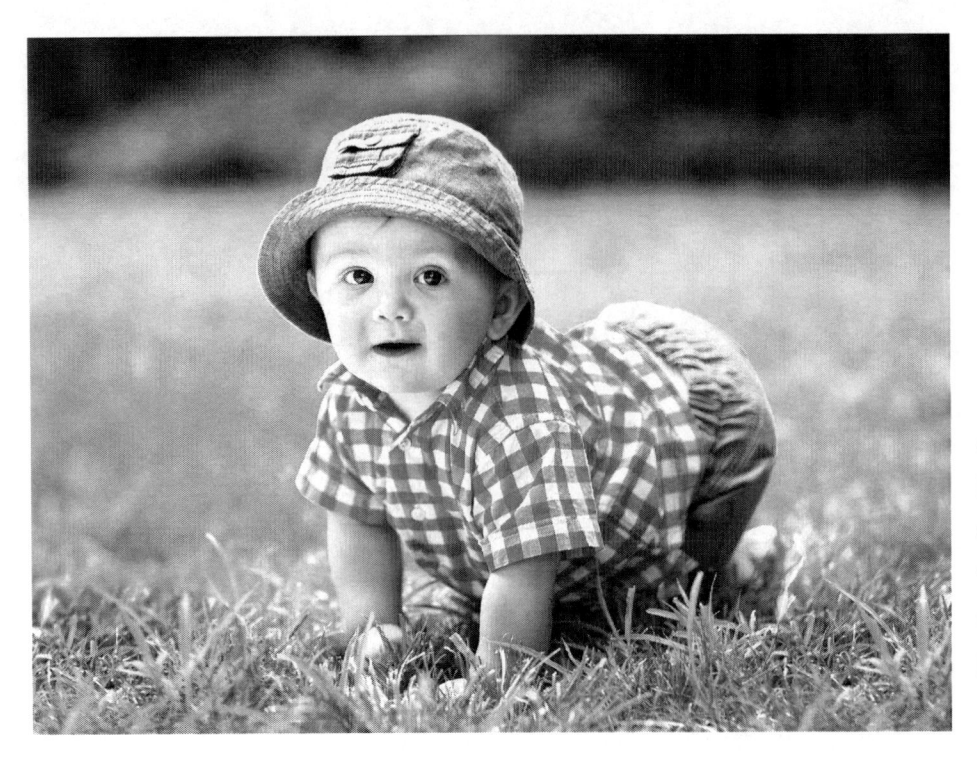

Children should have as much stimulation and freedom of movement as possible.

The systematic-exposure-to-movement tasks must be consistent with the child's developmental level. If a task is presented before the child is developmentally ready for it, the results will be unskilled performance or failure. Children introduced to tasks before they are developmentally ready are no better off (in fact, may be worse off) than those who learn tasks when they're fully prepared. If you attempt to teach children to walk prematurely, they may not develop movement skills usually learned with crawling. In addition, crawling develops muscle strength that is essential to maintaining balance in a standing position. The concept of readiness is based upon the normal developmental changes that occur during childhood.

The Child's Changing Body

Children grow at different rates. Individual differences in growth rates make it difficult to predict absolutely a child's readiness to learn skills. However, all children follow general growth patterns. A baby at birth is approximately one-fourth of his adult height. During the first three years after birth, the child grows rapidly in both height and weight. Growth rates are less rapid during the rest of childhood, continuing slowly and not as dramatically as before. At puberty, the time of the onset of sexual development, children grow rapidly again.

Body proportions change tremendously during childhood, and should be considered when analyzing and developing your child's exercise program. At birth, the head is disproportionably larger than the rest of the body, already having reached over 50 percent of its adult size. Neck muscles are relatively weak in babies, so it's important to support the head in certain exercises during the first years of life. There are specific exercises that will strengthen your child's neck muscles. During the first year after birth, the trunk is the fastest growing body segment, accounting for over 60 percent of the total increase in height. The legs are the fastest growing segment from about one year to the beginning of puberty. Late maturers generally have somewhat longer arms and legs than children who entered puberty earlier.

During childhood, girls and boys are usually about the same height and weight. However, girls are more mature at any given age, so they are closer to their adult height. Girls can usually be introduced to new motor skills earlier than boys because they are more mature and ready to learn sports movements.

Height increases are almost entirely due to growth of the skeleton. The skeleton undergoes profound changes during infancy. At birth, the bones are largely composed of cartilage, a soft pliable tissue. As the child grows, most of this cartilage is replaced by bone. Long-bone (leg and arm) formation occurs at the growth plates (sometimes called epiphyseal plates), located near the ends of long bones. Care must be taken to protect these bone growth centers during childhood. Too much throwing or regular heavy weight lifting can cause growth plate injuries that could be serious. Growth stops when the growth plates fuse.

Muscle growth is considerable between the first and seventh years but slows down in the years before puberty. Most of the increase in muscle size occurs from increases in muscle fiber size, a process called hypertrophy., During childhood, however, the number of muscle fibers also increases in a process called hyperplasia. The contribution of hyperplasia to muscle growth is probably minimal in most children. But the ability to promote an increase in the number of muscle fibers may have profound implications for young athletes heading for world-class performance. At present, researchers do not know what effect, if any, training during childhood has on hyperplasia. In adults, hypertrophy accounts for increases in muscle size.

During infancy and childhood there is a steady increase in the child's ability to make faster, more powerful movements. Although the development of fast-twitch muscles occurs before and during the first few months of life, these fibers cannot contract rapidly in the young child because the nervous system is still immature. You should consider the muscle contraction characteristics of children when you're trying to plan appropriate exercise experiences. Young children have difficulty performing fast movements, so premature exposure to sports that require fast movements or a lot of power in coordinated movements will be a waste of time until the child is five or six years old. Tennis is a good example—young children do not have the neuromuscular development to master the sport until later childhood.

The cardiovascular system performs remarkably well from the beginning of life. Before birth, the child is completely dependent upon gas and nutrient exchange in the enclosed maternal environment. After birth, the lungs take over and supply life-support functions. Young children have a great potential for performing endurance exercise without danger to their cardiovascular systems—in fact, five-year-olds have completed 26-mile marathons without ill effects. Continuous serious training in endurance running may not be a good idea for young children, however. Studies of animals suggest that excessive running during childhood may affect the growth centers of long bones. Extensive endurance training during this period could curtail the time in which important movement skills should be developing, and could result in psychological damage as well. Prolonged endurance exercise is not a natural part of normal play during childhood, although it is not known whether this phenomenon is biological or sociological in origin.

The ability to regulate body temperature is not fully developed in infants and young children. Great care must be afforded the physical comfort of young children in adverse environmental conditions. In the cold, clothing that might be adequate for the adult may not be enough for the child. However, young children are at a disadvantage if they wear too much clothing in the cold. Children adjust to heat because they have a large skin area compared to their muscle mass, which allows them to more easily dissipate heat from their bodies. In the heat, great care must be given to maintaining adequate water intake. Water is the best defense against heat stress and should be given freely. You may encounter ignorant coaches who withhold water from young children to "toughen them up." Don't stand for this—withholding water from children is negligent behavior.

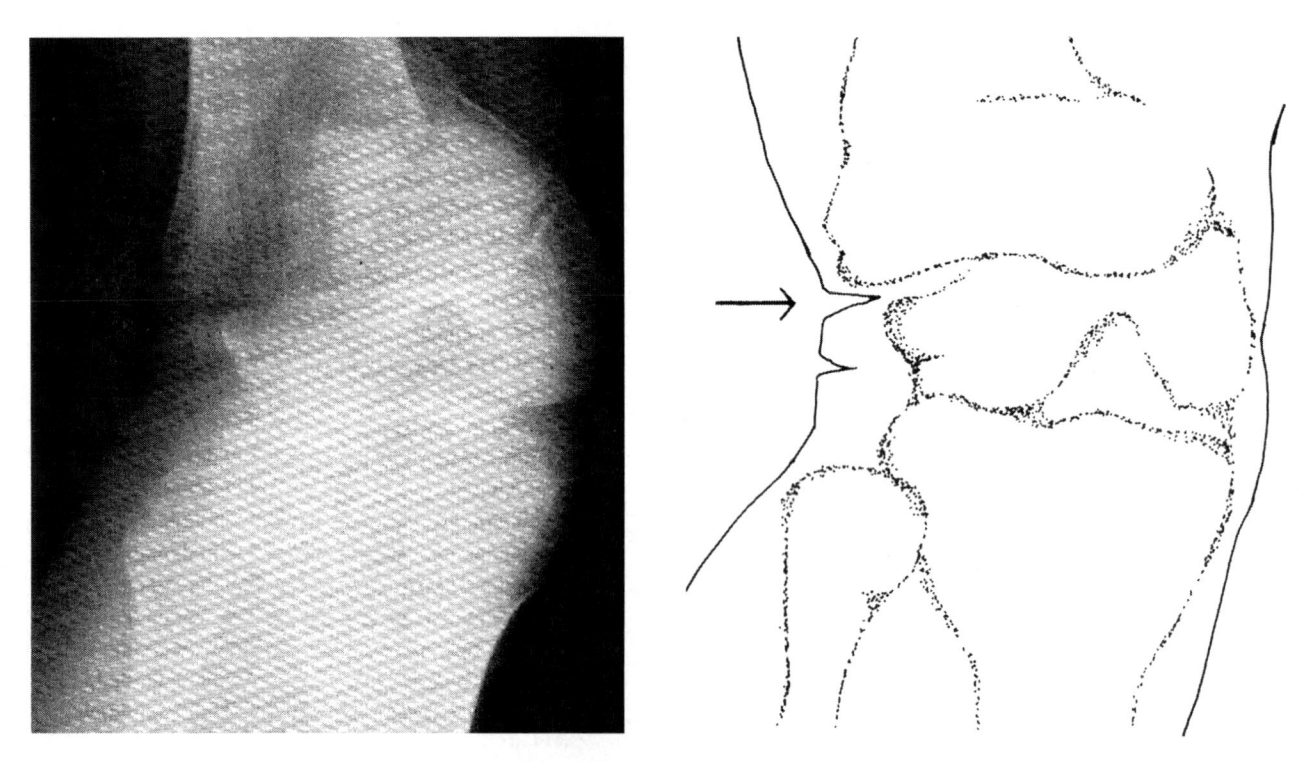

X-ray of a young girl's left knee shows separation of the growth plate (indicated by arrow), an epiphyseal injury which can hamper normal development of the bones.

Motor Development During Infancy

When you are trying to determine children's' readiness for sports, note how well they have mastered the basic movement skills. It's not a good idea to expect children to follow a precise developmental timetable, but you can make certain generalizations.

Obviously, babies move before they are born. (Sometimes it seems as though the unborn child is training a few rounds on a punching bag.) Pre-birth movements are related to vigor and movement potential after birth. Maternal exercise during pregnancy also affects the unborn baby—usually in the same way it affects the mother: The heart rates of mother and fetus increase, and the tissue of both have less oxygen, which stimulates an increased cardiovascular capacity. The long-range effects of training that occur in the mother also happen in the unborn child. The hearts of babies whose mothers exercised during pregnancy are larger, stronger, and have a greater capacity to pump blood. As you can see, preparing for optimal development begins even before birth.

At birth, the baby's movements are reflexes—physical responses not controlled by the brain. Some developmental experts think these reflexes serve as the basis for fundamental movement patterns that develop later. For example, infants held in an upright position will make walking movements. Another early movement pattern is the swimming reflex that occurs when the infant is immersed in water. Stimulating these early reflex patterns may affect later movement behavior.

During the first few months, children gain some head mobility and begin to watch objects with their eyes. After two months, children begin to respond to stimuli, such as smiling when parents smile at them. Even at this early age, parents can take advantage of the increase in perceptual ability to help children learn about their new environment by hanging mobiles over the crib or changing table and giving them rattles and different shaped objects.

By about four or five months, infants can make large muscle movements, such as pushing the body up with the arms when lying down. Children can also grasp objects. At this time, you can help children develop hand/eye coordination. They begin to discriminate between different sounds and the meaning of particular voice tones—the beginnings of perceptual skills important in sports.

Creeping, forward motion powered by the arms, usually begins by the sixth or seventh month. Crawling follows this movement. Around the ninth month, children can stand if supported. By the first year, they can walk if supported. The progression from creeping to crawling to upright support and then supported walking is important. Trying to speed up the development is futile and will deprive the child of valuable movement experiences. For example, crawling develops the back and abdominal strength that is necessary for walking.

By the beginning of the second year, most children have begun to walk. All children are different—some walk earlier than others. Don't become overanxious if your child isn't walking exactly at this time; prediction of movement development is only approximate.

Movement Exercises During Infancy

During the first year, the child should be given the maximum opportunity to develop a strong perception of the outside world. These opportunities can't be left to chance—parents must present novel tasks and situations for the infant to master and adapt to. Movement and perceptual facilitation is not a matter of forcing infants to be active, but one of giving them the opportunity for activity. If movement experiences are positive and occur in an atmosphere of love and care, then the baby will want to repeat these experiences often, which will develop movement skills.

The development of skilled movements progresses from a series of basic experiences. Newborns have had few experiences other than those in the aqueous environment of the womb. Infants should be exposed to a variety of perceptual and motor experiences beginning the first few days of life. One of the most important of these for perceptual and motor development is human contact. The baby learns to react to stimulation by the parent and, in the process, develops the senses. Human contact should be restricted to a few people during the first week or two. Too many people may over stimulate the child and adversely affect perceptual development.

Early perceptual and motor training involves providing maximum opportunity for the baby's involvement with the environment. Bright colored objects held within the view of a new baby will eventually attract his or her attention. After the infant learns to focus on an object, you can slowly move it and attempt to have the baby track it with his eyes. As the baby's ability to watch objects increases, you can make movements more complex by requiring head movements in a variety of directions. After five months of exposure to these exercises, the baby will have developed some of the basic movement and perceptual skills that will later prove indispensable in learning complex skills, such as catching a ball.

Kinesthesis, the ability to recognize body positions, can also be developed early. During the first weeks after birth, babies learn new things about their new environment every time you hold them in a different position. At first, this involves simply supporting the baby on one arm and then the other. As the baby grows, try holding him on his side, on his back, up in the air, and eventually upside down.

Proprioception can be developed in water. Partially immersing your baby in warm water will stimulate movement (the swimming reflex) and improve perception. Infants have an active swimming reflex, which enables them to make coordinated swimming movements until they are four months old, when the reflex disappears. Critics argue that actual swimming skills are not maintained and actually deteriorate during infancy. However, moving in water does seem to improve perceptual facilities and helps engender an adventuresome spirit in young children. You might want to enroll your child in a swimming program for infants. Timidness and fear are prevalent in children with limited experience. Enjoyable, positive experiences create an environment for further learning and exploration.

Exercises to develop hand/eye coordination can also begin in infancy. Suspend an object near the baby; he or she will eventually come in contact with it by chance. After repeated

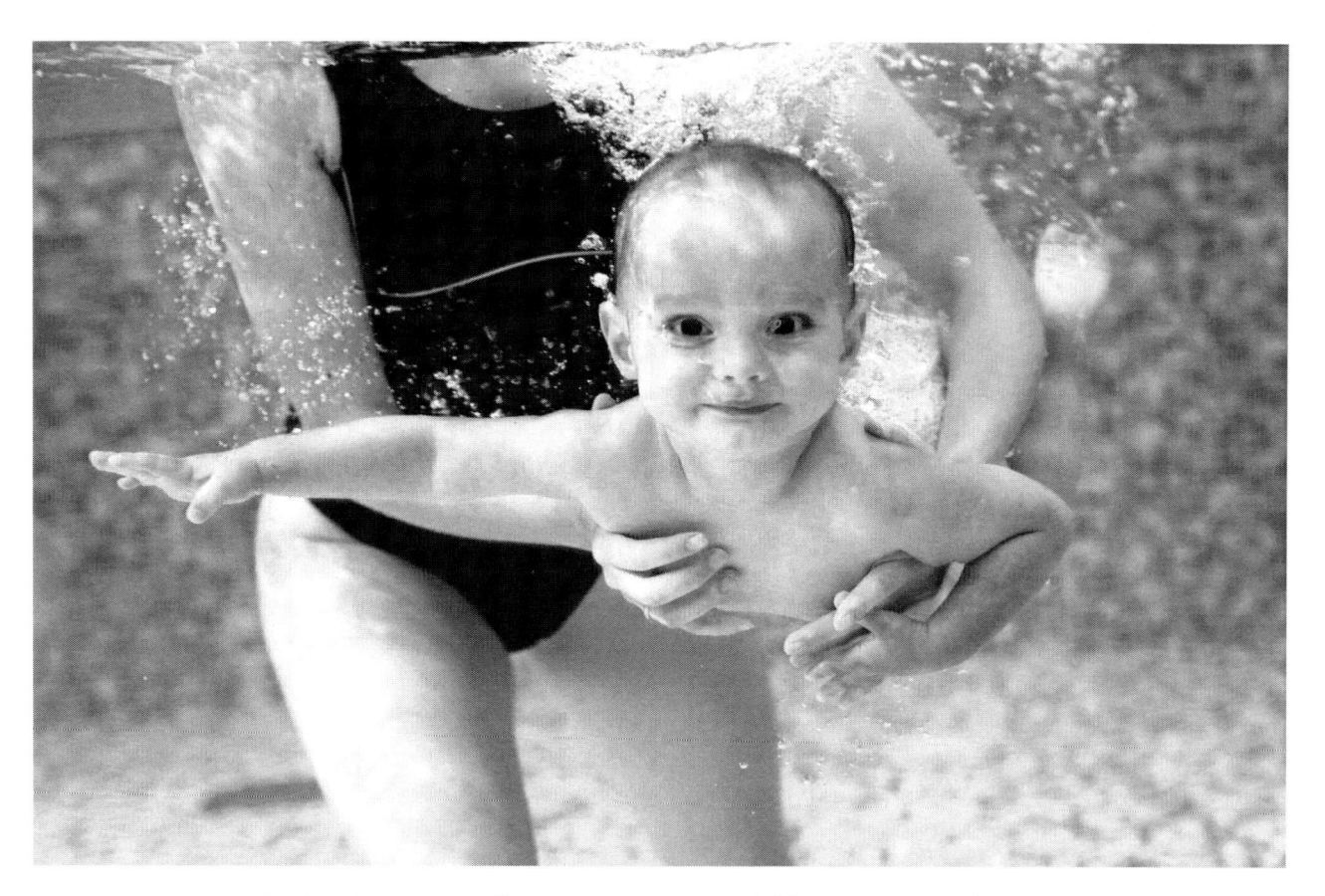

Moving in water will improve a young child's perceptual facilities and engender an adventuresome spirit.

encounters with random items, the baby will reach for the items purposely. As the baby's competence increases, gradually make the tasks more varied and complex; for example, try getting the baby to grasp a moving object. The next step might be to move the object in different directions. Later, you can make noises while you stimulate your child to visually track and grab for an object, thereby combining several senses at once and working on simultaneous coordination of sight, sound, and movement. There are literally thousands of exercises you can perform with newborn infants to improve their senses. Use a little imagination.

An important aspect of the perceptual-motor development of infants involves whole-body movements. In general, try to allow the greatest possible amount of movement consistent, of course, with the safety of the child and the rights of others. Infants should wear as little clothing as possible. Binding clothing restricts movement and makes them uncomfortable. If the room is warm enough (above 75 degrees), babies will not have to wear too much clothing; they will be comfortable and capable of movement with only a minimum of restrictions.

By the fourth to sixth month, you can place your baby in a variety of situations to help develop whole-body movements. At first, place the baby on her belly and encourage her

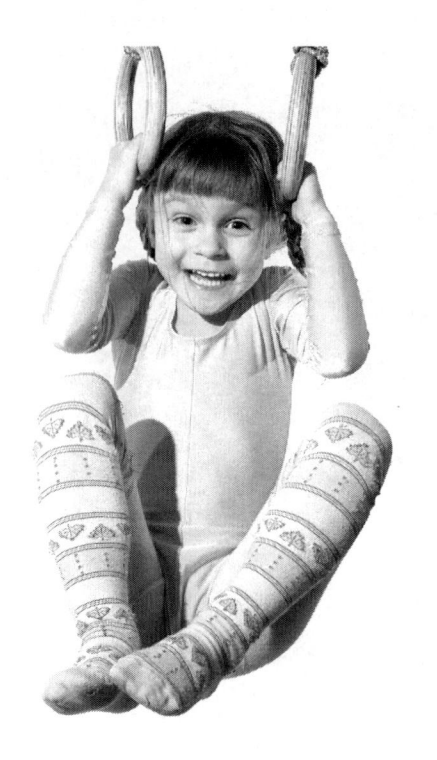

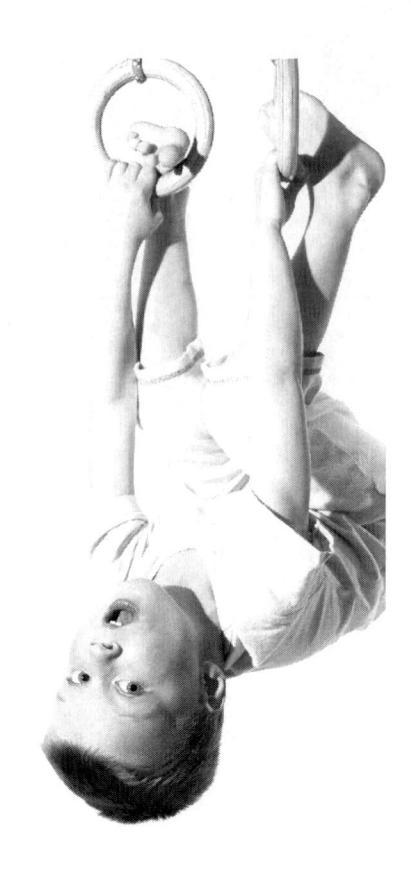

Kindergyms provide experiences through "structured play" in a completely non-competitive environment.

to reach for objects. Then you can combine exercises involving visual and grasping abilities by encouraging the baby, when he is on his back, to grasp a ring or stick and pull himself up.

Beginning in about the fourth month, children should have increasing exposure to a variety of people. There are structured motor development programs, called kindergyms or babygyms, available throughout the country. In addition to providing an opportunity for movement, these programs serve as an introduction to socialization with other children. Socialization skills are important, too, for optimal development. These programs stress movement experiences and are completely non-competitive. They provide "structured play"—children can climb and play on the trampoline, balance beam, monkey bars and trapeze. They are valuable for children as young as five or six months and as old as ten or twelve years.

Beginning at about month five, babies can play in jumpers. These are harness and spring devices suspended from a frame or the ceiling. Infants' feet barely touch the floor as they sit in the jumper; but they can jump up and down freely. The jumper is great for developing back and leg muscles and proprioception. Start off with short bouts of about one to three minutes, then gradually increase the amount of time in the jumper, up to about five minutes.

As the baby begins to creep and crawl, at about month seven, you can work on developing his or her mobility skills in a variety of ways. Encourage the baby to crawl under and over objects, move on irregular surfaces, and climb up steps. Let your child walk naturally. Devices such as walkers don't develop the skills and strengths required in walking and are of little value. Creeping and crawling skills should be fully mastered as they serve as important prerequisites to later motor development.

When your child begins to stand, you can certainly help by providing encouragement and maximum opportunity to walk. As the child begins to walk, try to develop this new movement capability in a variety of ways. At first, encourage the child to walk longer distances. Then expose him or her to different surfaces, such as sand, pebbles, irregular surfaces, side-facing slopes, inclines, declines, and stairs. Continue to offer more difficult tasks to further improve walking skills. Have the child walk the length of a board; then raise the board off the ground with blocks and have him try it. Have the child carry objects while walking. As walking skills improve, teach the child to kick a ball. Let him watch you do it or simply put a ball in front of his feet when he's standing.

Motor Development During Childhood

After learning to walk, a child's world becomes larger. The first years of greater mobility are extremely important for developing the basic movements that will determine success in sports skills. During this time, it's easy to become complacent because the child seems so active. Why, you might ask, is more systematic activity important? Because it's vital that movement skills be learned in progression—the child must work to improve.

Improvement during infancy was a matter of providing constructive opportunities for movement. The infant was given many chances for trial-and-error learning experiences. During childhood, chance exposures to movement become less important, and instruction becomes necessary for maximum skill development. To be sure, there should always be a trial-and-error component to learning, but children should also have the opportunity to learn by example. They need models to develop such complex motor skills as throwing and catching.

Don't over intellectualize with children. Demonstrate the skill and then let them learn it by trial and error. Most kids don't profit from verbal instruction. One of the most ridiculous scenes I've ever observed occurred at a Lake Tahoe ski resort during a children's ski lesson:

"Now, Sally, I want you to traverse the hill with your weight on your downhill ski. Keep your uphill shoulder forward and your hands in front of you. When you are ready to turn, take your weight off the edges and your skis will naturally go down the hill. Then put the weight on the inside edge of your outer ski—because of the curvature of your skis, they will turn naturally."

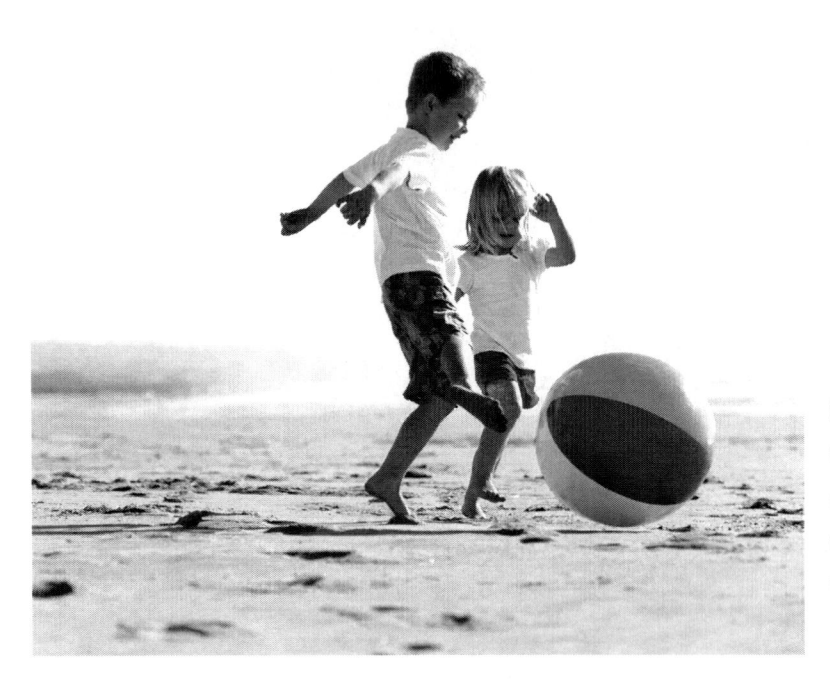

Encourage your child to walk and play on different surfaces and become familiar with them.

Sally was a five-year-old child who had been skiing for about five or six days. She looked at her instructor as though he were speaking Latin. It's counterproductive to intellectualize sports technique with children—for that matter, it may not even be a good idea with adults. A child must learn to perform coordinated movements automatically. Coordination occurs more through "body learning" than through "mind learning." You create efficient movements by gradually eliminating unproductive movements. Most sports teachers who specialize in teaching children emphasize imitation and games that cause children to assume proper movement patterns. Children's ski schools at Buttermilk in Aspen and Squaw Valley in Lake Tahoe pattern their programs on the developmental characteristics of the kids. They teach by example and by structured trial-and-error experimentation.

During childhood, skill development depends mostly upon increasing proficiency in basic skills already learned, and so it's very important to provide plenty of experience at each stage of learning. For example, if a child doesn't receive enough practice in visual tracking during early childhood, it may be extremely difficult for the child at seven or eight to hit a softball. Make sure your child gets a chance to systematically develop these basic movement and perceptual skills:

- Walking and Running
- Jumping, Hopping, Skipping, and Galloping
- Climbing
- Body Image
- Balancing
- Throwing and Catching
- Dynamic Vision

Walking and Running

Although children begin to walk a little after their first birthday, they don't master balance until much later. Children begin walking with a relatively wide stance. Until a child is older than two years, walking is visually monitored—very young children have difficulty "feeling" their bodies. At about eighteen months, the child begins a fast walk. This is not a true run because both feet never leave the ground simultaneously. The child begins true forward running between the second and third years, and gradually develops the ability to run to the side (lateral mobility) and backwards. The child learns to stop and start rapidly at about four or five years of age. Running has many component skills: moving to the left and right; stopping and starting; varying speed; and maintaining speed when assuming different balancing positions (running under a low overhand, for example). The child should have practice in the various aspects of running. Running skills are fundamental to efficient sports performance.

Jumping, Hopping, Skipping, and Galloping

Children begin jumping at about one and a half years, when they can step off a low step. Jumping progresses from one-foot to two-foot takeoffs. Most children develop good jumping skills by the time they're four or five years old. Hopping, skipping, and galloping—skills similar to jumping—are also developed during early childhood. Social forces affect the learning of these skills; boys better develop galloping and girls better master skipping.

Children exhibit gender differences in play preference as early as infancy and are at least partially due to subtle social pressures. Even today in our activity-oriented society there is different movement emphasis for each gender. Girls are often encouraged to play in an orderly fashion and participate in activities such as dance and gymnastics. Boys are taught not to skip and are steered away from so-called feminine activities in favor of developing basic sports skills, such as throwing, catching, running, and jumping. Both boys and girls are cheated out of valuable movement experiences because of these restrictive social attitudes.

Climbing

The development of the climbing skill begins even before the child walks. Children will attempt to climb ladders before they are one-year old, if given the opportunity. Climbing requires a combination of upper and lower body coordination and daring. Bravery and daring are traits difficult to measure, but they play an important role in the acquisition and development of movement skills. These traits depend on the degree of self-assuredness the child has; self-assuredness, in turn, depends on a series of successes and a variety of experiences. Climbing does subject the child to a certain amount of physical risk. However, skill development under somewhat adverse conditions will make the child more competent to deal with similar situations in the future. Fear develops because of uncertainty in the face of the unknown or the dangerous. Children who develop a variety of motor skills will have a wide repertoire of options available in dangerous or challenging situations. Encourage activities such as climbing, crawling, and hanging. You can watch your child closely during these movements to make sure he or she doesn't get hurt. The movement skill gained far outweighs the relative danger involved.

Body image—the awareness of body parts and their movement potential—is extremely important for the development of movement skills and a positive self-image. The development of this trait follows two tracks—intuitive recognition of the body and its parts, and verbal identification and recognition. Intuitive recognition develops earlier than verbal identification. By about age four, most children can point out major body parts, such as the head, tummy, legs, elbows, and shoulders, when they are called out.

Children use a variety of movements when they attempt a task. One week the child may display tremendous progress in learning a skill; the next week he or she appears to be starting all over again. The inconsistency exhibited can be maddening to the parent. The child doesn't really regress, however; he is only working on a different aspect of learning the movement. The ability to vary technique is important to develop body image fully. The parent, therefore, should not necessarily intervene when the child seems to be regressing. The important thing is to provide the maximum number of opportunities for experimentation and practice. Accurate assessment of the child's capabilities is not really possible until the child is between seven and eleven years old.

Laterality, a skill associated with body image, is not fully developed until eight to eleven years of age. This skill is the ability to differentiate between and move to the left or the right. It is a later basic skill, extremely important for sports techniques. Unfortunately, it is often lacking in the adult, perhaps because its development occurs at a time when many children get turned off about movement or at a time when other basic skills have not been learned as they should have been. Don't let this be the beginning of a cycle of failure for your child. Keep working to make movement experiences positive and successful.

Balancing

Balance skills progress rapidly after children learn to stand. By three years of age, a child can usually walk the length of a narrow ten-foot line. By five, children can stand on one foot for several seconds. Girls are usually superior to boys in balance skills at any given age during childhood.

Children can learn recreational balance sports, such as snow boarding, water skiing, surfing, and skateboarding at about five years of age. Before this time, children lack the muscle strength and moving balance ability to learn these sports. However, exposure to snow skiing before balancing skills are fully developed may be valuable for children; it can help them gain familiarity with wearing skis during walking movements and simple glides. Skilled turns will take a little more maturity.

Throwing and Catching

Throwing is a basic skill that is extremely important for success in many sports. Several developmental levels characterize throwing skills. Children go through several developmental levels when learning to throw a ball. They will have difficulty fully developing throwing skills if they don't fully master each level. Throwing patterns in the two-year-old involve the arm and shoulder only, and the child often has better success throwing with an underhand motion. The next developmental phase involves turning the trunk, but the arm and shoulders are still the most important factor in generating power in the throw. At about four years, the child begins to use more of a sidearm motion with more trunk rotation. At five or six, the child begins to shift body weight when throwing. The final throwing stage involves stepping in the direction of the ball, in addition to trunk rotation and slight sidearm motion. This mature throwing pattern allows the child to exert maximum force.

Girls often fail to develop mature throwing techniques. This is probably a sociological phenomenon that reflects lack of long-term practice rather than a true ability difference. If you encourage and instruct your daughter through the various phases, there is no reason why she shouldn't develop full power throwing techniques.

Catching skills are also very important for success in sports. These skills are more difficult to master than throwing skills because catching requires many basic sensory and movement abilities, such as hand/eye coordination, proprioception, and the ability to react and move rapidly. In addition, catching an object is never quite the same task two times in a row—if a ball is thrown at a different speed or to a slightly different spot, then the child must react in slightly different ways. In early attempts at catching, children usually hold out their hands with arms straight. Gradually, they learn to grasp with the hands while bending the elbows to absorb the force of the thrown object. At first, children have much better luck catching balls they have thrown themselves. At about five years of age, a child can catch a six-inch rubber playground ball if it is bounced to him from a short distance. Coordinated catching skills are not developed until at least ten years of age, and require a lot of practice to master.

The limiting factors in developing catching ability include visual tracking and visual perception. Until adolescence, a child doesn't have full ability to judge the speed of a rapidly moving object and determine the necessary position to catch it. The visual perception necessary in sports takes a lot of practice for a child to develop.

Skill Refinement

The period between six and twelve years old is extremely important for the integration of basic movement skills into sports games. During this period of refinement of basic skills, some youngsters are escalated into a lifetime of physical activity while others are left by the wayside. During later childhood, movement skills become more specific—success in one skill will not necessarily mean success in another. The specificity of tasks is based largely on the increased complexity of movements practiced by the older child. The movements of all infants, for example, are similar and usually develop around the same time. Movements in older children, however, are based on years of cumulative experiences that are unique to each child. While walking is an instinctive behavior, hitting a forehand or skiing is not. Skilled movements require practice.

All of the physical abilities mentioned above continue to increase in both boys and girls until the beginning of puberty. The improvements in skills are due to an increased maturity of the nervous system and increased strength. Toward the end of childhood, girls generally start to level off in their ability to jump, run, and throw. Girls, however, continue to be as good or better than boys in the ability to balance and hop—two skills that are often important parts of play among girls. Girls also exceed boys in some' agility and rhythmical activities.

Movement and Sports Exercises During Childhood

During early childhood, the focus should be on developing such basic movement skills as walking, balancing, throwing, and catching. This early practice should involve both specific drills and integration of basic skills into unstructured games and play. As the child moves into middle and late childhood, introduce more structured games and sports.

Formal conditioning exercises, such as running laps around a track or specific callisthenic exercises, should not begin until the child reaches school age. During the elementary school years, children can engage in vigorous physical activity but shouldn't be subjected to the rigors of structured running and swimming regimens. It's critical that basic skills and sports fundamentals be stressed over high levels of conditioning and advanced sports tactics. Premature emphasis on conditioning and tactics diminishes enjoyment of movement and curtails time that should be spent on basic skills.

Structured athletic programs are not bad during childhood. However, these programs should stress learning skills rather than competition. I've observed summer baseball leagues for young children that spend more time on championship playoff games than on the round robin games of the regular schedule. It's much more important to let a lot of kids play throughout the summer than to narrow the participation down to a few "all-stars." This kind of athletic structure can't possibly be for the good of the child.

Developing Walking Skills

There is no abrupt transition when the child goes from crawling to walking. During the first stages of walking, a child may prefer crawling at times because it's still a faster way to move. Give your child the maximum opportunity for movement under whatever mode of travel he or she prefers.

As the child increases the amount of walking, encourage full development of these skills. Begin by getting him to walk farther. Stand at increasing distances from the child and encourage him to come to you. Put objects such as chairs in his path so he must go around them to get to his destination. Give him the opportunity to crawl and walk up stairs and on irregular surfaces, such as grass, sand, snow, pebbles, and dirt. Let him try to walk on slanted surfaces—the beach would be perfect for this. Have him walk while carrying objects; then have him avoid obstacles in his path while carrying the objects.

Developing Running Skills and Cardiovascular Endurance

The transition from walking to running is gradual. It begins with a fast walk. As balance and leg strength improve, the child learns to run. There are many variables associated with running skills. Spontaneous running in a straight line is easier than the stop-and-start or lateral running required in soccer, or even in the games children make up themselves.

It's important that running be a pleasurable experience for the child from the beginning. Running is the best exercise for developing cardiovascular fitness for people at any age. For the adult, running provides a means of getting a good workout in a relatively short period of time. Parents can set a good example by running regularly and including the child in family runs. Children can begin participating in family fun runs at about three years of age. Don't force the child to run; just provide the opportunity to be included in an enjoyable family activity. Family exercise outings can also be used as an opportunity to monitor your child's progress. Set up short races and obstacle courses. If they are carried out in a spirit of fun, the child will get a chance to develop healthy competitiveness in an atmosphere of fun and support. You can encourage your child to improve his or her running times and instill the idea of self-improvement.

Games play an important part of developing endurance and running skills during childhood. Soccer is probably the best-structured sport for children as preparation for sports participation in later years because it develops many basic skills. Even future football player would profit from playing soccer during childhood. Football skills can be learned during adolescence; but the same cannot be said for the basic movement skills that soccer teaches. In general, try to get your child to participate in sports that involve considerable activity. The six-year-old girl who stands idle in center field is not getting enough exposure to vital running skills.

Cardiovascular endurance is improved by exercising harder for a longer time periods. Sports scientists have determined that the best exercises for developing endurance include those requiring the rhythmical use of large muscle areas for long time durations. Specific examples include running and walking, swimming, bicycling, and cross-country skiing. Although you can introduce these activities during childhood, serious training should be delayed until the child is at least eight to ten years of age.

Developing Balance and Proprioception

Because running and walking require balance, balance is effectively developed while the child practices these skills. There are many kinds of balance, so practicing a variety of activities best develops balance.

Riding a bicycle is a balance task that practically all children are anxious to master. A child can best begin to learn cycling skills on a tricycle, which teaches the basic movement patterns required in cycling. Next the child can progress to a bicycle with training wheels (auxiliary small wheels attached to the rear wheel of the bike). All children do not need training wheels; however, for most kids, the use of these supports will accelerate progress. After the child has mastered cycling with the training wheels, let him or her try riding without them. You can run along side to prevent a serious crash. If the child has practiced enough with the training wheels, mastering two-wheel cycling should not be difficult.

Skateboarding, rollerblading, and snowboarding are great ways to develop balance skills. Although children younger than five won't become very skillful, merely standing and walking on skates or skis will contribute to their balance skills. Be careful not to push or frighten children-keep these early experiences positive. Watch out for the safety of children, and be sure they wear protective equipment. Skateboarding and roller-skating require, a helmet, kneepads, and elbow pads. Check to make sure that the ski bindings young skiers use work properly.

Stilts, bongo boards (a board balanced on a cylinder), and pogo sticks are used by school-age children to advance balance skills, although these devices require good body control and balance skills that are fairly well developed. The trampoline is a good way to teach children to balance their body when they're moving. The trampoline helps children "feel" their body in a three-dimensional space (proprioception). This device is losing popularity in schools across the country because of liability problems. Serious spinal injuries have occurred when children did certain kinds of somersaults on the trampoline. This is unfortunate because trampolines can be excellent devices for developing balance, proprioception, and muscle strength in children older than two or three. If used properly, they are safe. Trampolines can be purchased from various gymnastics equipment manufacturers, and most recreational departments and gymnastics clubs have them. An alternative to a trampoline is an old spring mattress; children can bounce on it and learn to control their bodies when they're thrown off balance.

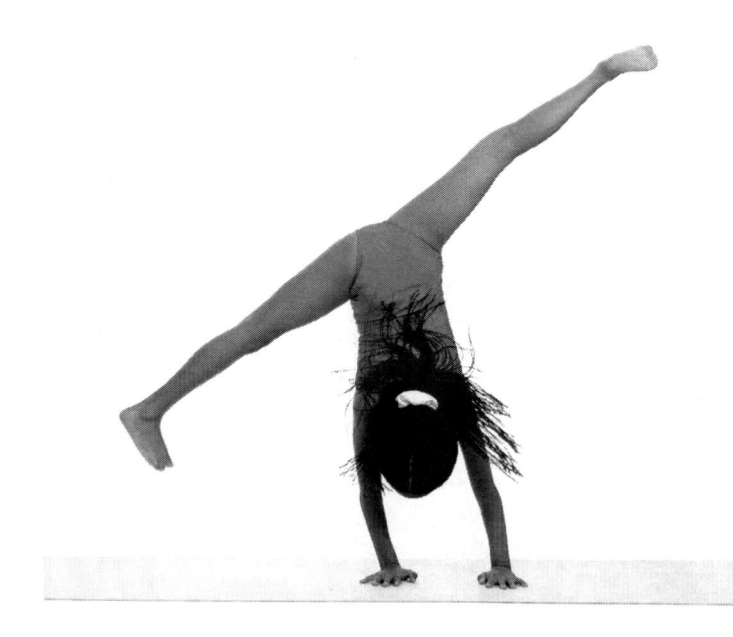

Tumbling allows a child to master body movements and develop complex sports skills like balance and proprioception.

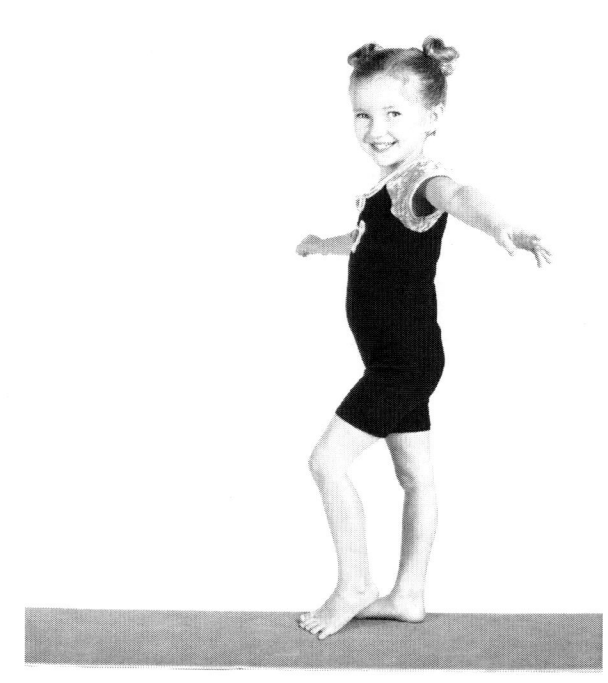

Walking on the balance beam allows a child to feel his body in a three-dimensional space (proprioception).

Gymnastics skills such as tumbling, walking on the balance beam, and working with a gymnastics harness can also contribute to the development of balance and proprioception. These exercises can begin at two years of age. Somersaults, cartwheels, and headstands teach children to master their bodies and serve as the basis for many other sports skills. If the gymnastics harness is used as a swing, it can give children a chance to experience the sensation of speed. The harness can also be used to allow children to perform gymnastics maneuvers such as flips safely.

Climbing is important for developing whole-body coordination, strength, balance, and an adventuresome spirit. This skill should be developed early. Children can learn to climb up a ladder even before they can walk. Climbing tasks are important for helping the child gain the strength to handle his or her own body, a prerequisite for many sports skills.

Developing Coordination in Children

Coordination is the efficient use of perceptual and motor abilities in the performance of a physical task. There is no separate skill called coordination. A coordinated person has many specific abilities and skills which he or she applies automatically and efficiently to a particular situation. The person is, therefore, able to adjust physically to any circumstances. Movement experiences involving perceptual and motor skills contribute to coordination.

A good activity for developing coordination, endurance, strength, and balance is jumping rope. You can usually introduce this task when the child is about three and a half years old. Initially, hold the rope three to six inches from the ground and have the child jump over it. Get the child used to jumping over the rope at various heights. Next, have two people each hold an end of the rope; move the rope from

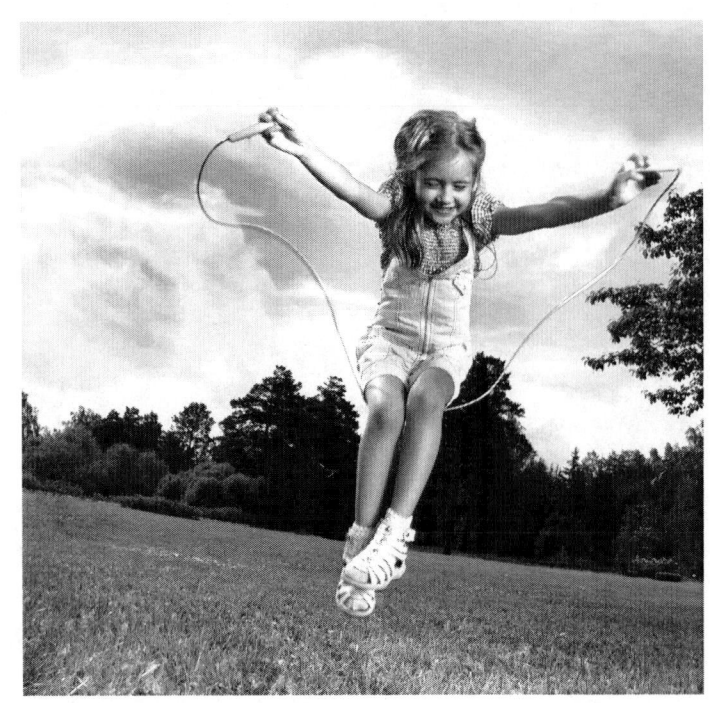

Jumping rope can acquaint children with spacial awareness and rhythm.

side to side and have the child jump as the rope approaches. Gradually, get the child to increase the number of times he or she can jump in succession. As the child becomes more skilled, circle the rope completely over his or her head. During the early phases of learning this skill, the child will make a small jump between jumps over the rope. This seems to help rhythm and allows time to prepare for the next big jump. As jump-roping skills become proficient, teach the child to hold the rope and turn it.

Rope skipping is generally more popular among girls than boys, who often think it's feminine. But show a young boy a picture of a boxer, such as Muhammad Ali, skipping rope and you will quickly dispel this notion.

Another good way to develop coordination, muscle strength, and flexibility is to exercise with a parachute. (You can buy a parachute at an Army surplus store.) Children enjoy the way the chute floats and undulates in the air. With the parachute, children can achieve a vigorous movement experience in a non-competitive environment. Have four to six people space themselves in a circle, grab the outer edge of the parachute, and lift their arms so that the chute fills with air. Once the chute is airborne, there are many vigorous movements children can do; these include touching their toes while holding the chute, running in a circle while holding the chute, and simply shaking the chute.

Perceptual and motor development depend upon a good sense of three-dimensional space. Manipulating objects and substances such as blocks and clay is important for developing hand/eye coordination and strength in the hands and forearms. These experiences can begin in infancy. Young children can also gain valuable experience by playing in the

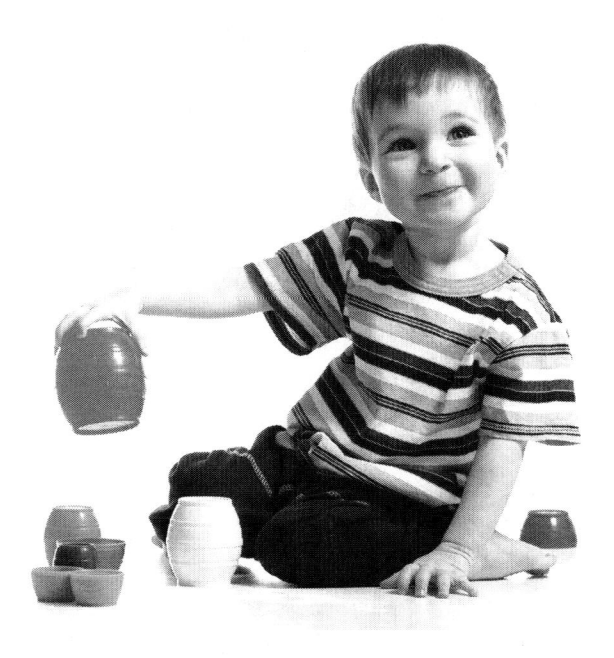

Blocks can help develop motor skills and coordination.

sand; show them how to turn wet sand into balls and sand castles. An old typewriter or computer keyboard can provide a young child the opportunity to develop finger dexterity that will be valuable in later sports. Games like marbles and jacks are good for children between four and ten years. Provide children with activities as drawing, hammering, and painting, where they can see the effects of work done with the hands. Activities like these provide the link between the sensory and motor systems.

Children should have a lot of experience playing on playground equipment, such as monkey bars, rings, and geometrical shapes. These structures allow children to develop spatial awareness in addition to strength and whole-body movement skills. They also give children a chance to develop body image—knowledge of what their bodies are capable of doing. You can construct monkey bars out of pipes from a hardware store, and many playgrounds have a variety of geometrical shapes for children to climb on.

Children love to move to music. Use music early to stimulate movement in children. Start dancing to music and even a very young child will join in and imitate you. Music increases enthusiasm for exercise and creates an atmosphere of fun.

Coordinated movements require a well-developed body image. Children need an intuitive knowledge of how their bodies perform skillful movements. You can help develop this knowledge by teaching children to identify different body parts verbally. Then help them identify and perform various movements—nodding or turning the head, bending the arm, bending the knees, pointing the toes, and shrugging the shoulders. First they can imitate you; then you can teach them to do the move-

GETTING OFF TO A FAST START | **49**

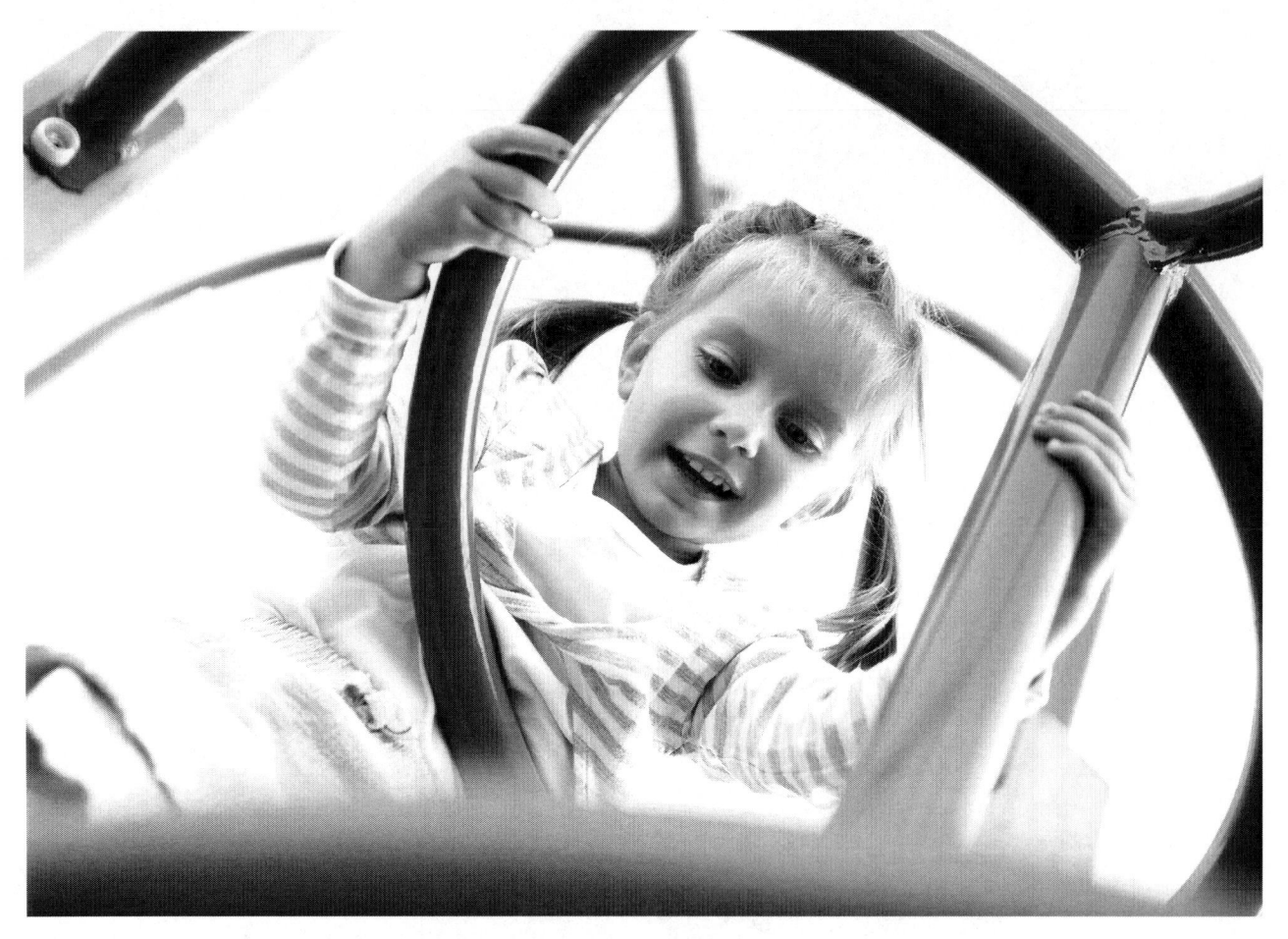

Playground equipment can help children develop spatial awareness, strength, and whole-body movement skills.

ment when you call it out. Work on developing laterality, the ability to move to the left and right. At first, play games that identify the left and right sides of the body; then try to develop the ability to move to the left or right. Determine the child's dominant side, the side that's strongest and used most. It is possible to have different dominant sides for hands and feet, so do upper and lower body movements. Work on developing the non-dominant side. For example, encourage a right-dominant child to hop on the left foot as well as the right, throw with the left hand, and run laterally to the left. Games like hopscotch are great for developing these skills if you encourage the child to use both the dominant and non-dominant sides. You can set up obstacle courses that require children to move to the left and right and jump up and down.

Homemade obstacle courses can help children develop such skills as running, agility, climbing, crawling, flexibility, spatial awareness, and body image, and develop a "movement library" that can later be drawn upon for skilled sports performances. Construct your obstacle course out of available materials and furniture: picnic benches, old tires, boxes, chairs, hula hoops, stairs, ropes, and whatever else you can think of.

Throwing and Catching

Throwing and catching are two of the most important and most difficult skills to master. These skills are used directly in sports like football, baseball, softball, and basketball, and indirectly in volleyball, tennis, badminton, lacrosse, and racquetball. The less physically mature children often do not get enough practice in these vital skills—ironically, of course, because they are the ones who need it most. Most elementary school physical education programs are directed at high achievers, who are usually the more mature children. Programs at the elementary level typically include structured games that demand basic throwing and catching skills; children who are good at these skills usually get to play more. The slower or less mature children get less game time and are often cheated out of valuable practice and instruction in the basic skills. There are some fine elementary school programs in this country, but, unfortunately, the majority of programs are a disgrace. Most are recess-type recreational programs that require survival of the fittest. To master such basic skills as throwing and catching, children must practice for many hours. Placing children prematurely in game situations do not effectively develop these skills.

Throwing skills begin to develop in infants when they accidentally release an object they happen to be flailing about. Keep a seven-inch rubber playground ball lying around so that your child gets used to handling a ball. As the child's ability grows, show him some movements he can perform with the ball. Have him

Complex ball-handling skills can only be developed through continual practice of basic throwing and catching.

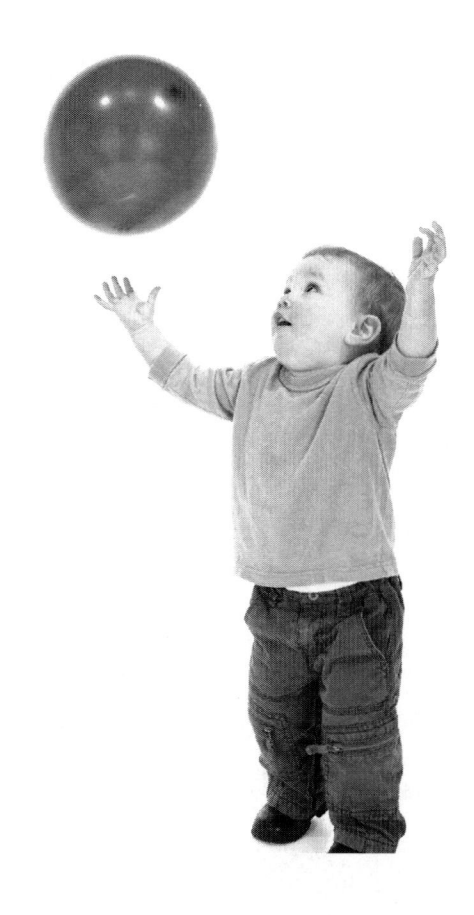

kick it—this will help balancing and running skills. Teach him to roll the ball—this will show him the ball's movement characteristics. Roll the ball to him and encourage him to stop it. You will probably have better luck with a young child if you use a smaller rubber ball to develop early throwing skills. The playground ball is best for developing catching skills.

You will find that the child will handle and catch a ball best if he throws it himself. At first, have him simply bounce the ball and catch it. Then add some variations: get him to throw the ball up and catch it; have the child throw and catch the ball while running. With just a little imagination, you will find many variations to this early ball-handling experience.

After a while, throwing and catching skills can be practiced with another person. Start by tossing the ball to your child underhand; then get your child to catch the ball from a bounce. Incorporate overhand throws and combinations of catching the ball from a bounce and from a fly.

Dribbling and hitting skills can be introduced as the child gains skill, usually at about six to eight years. Teach the child to bounce the ball with both hands, then with each hand separately. Show him how to bounce the ball and hit it like a baseball with his hand. As ball handling skills increase, children should perform these simple drills while running.

There are many auxiliary activities that help to develop ball-handling skills. A tetherball, which is a ball attached to a rope and pole, allows the child to track an object visually and make contact with it repeatedly. A punching bag provides similar practice; start off with a large punching bag that a child can easily handle. Another good practice device is the backstop, which looks like a small trampoline. The child throws a ball at the backstop and the ball bounces back.

Bean bags, Frisbees, balloons, and ring tosses each give children a chance to develop throwing and catching skills, and contribute to the development of hand/eye coordination.

As your child progresses and becomes more mature, make ball-handling tasks more challenging. At about eight to eleven years old, a child can begin working with a baseball, football, and basketball. It's important for the child to get concentrated practice in advanced ball handling before he or she incorporates these skills into game situations. Skilled sports performances are based on sound fundamentals, and the development of these fundamentals must follow the "three P's": practice, practice, and practice.

The Elementary-School Physical Education Program

Most resources in physical education are aimed at junior and senior high school students rather than the elementary level where it is needed most. High schools often have well-trained physical educators and extensive athletic facilities, while elementary schools usually have little more than token programs. Few programs have physical education specialists and most elementary school teachers receive little or no training in motor development and physical education. And in these days of shrinking educational budgets, elementary school physical education programs are often the first to go. Because of these circumstances, many children are cheated out of valuable and necessary developmental and educational experiences. Random play is not enough to develop movement skills adequately. Children who are slower or less mature than their playmates often will not get a chance to develop skills because they cannot perform up to the level of the more skillful.

The main purpose of the elementary school program should be to help children acquire a love of physical activity and help them develop basic motor and perceptual abilities, which they need to perform successfully in all movement environments. Emphasize balance, body and space awareness, hand/eye and foot/eye coordination, and running skills.

The ideal program should focus on:

- **Personalization.** Special consideration should be given to each child, including the normal, gifted, handicapped, poorly coordinated, and slow-learning child.

- **Love of Physical Activity.** They should learn that regular exercise is an important and enjoyable part of their day.

- **Development of efficient motor skills.** Children must learn how to run, jump, skip, climb, throw, and catch. Basic motor skills cannot be left to chance and should be systematically taught.

- **Development of perceptual-motor skills.** Children should develop perceptual abilities that are essential for general classroom learning as well as efficient movement. Teachers should identify children with special needs and help them overcome their perceptual motor deficiencies.

- **Sports and game skills.** After children have acquired the basic motor skills and feel confident about using their bodies, they need to be introduced to more specific instruction in game and sports activities. These activities should be progressively more challenging, but should emphasize the value of participation rather than winning or losing. Activities should include both individual and team sports, with emphasis placed on lifelong participation.

- **Positive self-image.** Children should develop a feeling of respect for the mind and body, along with confidence in their ability to function effectively in any situation. The physical education program should give each child a chance to improve and be active without having to live up to the expectations of others.

Put these ideas in action by modifying traditional games, such as kickball, that involve little exercise or skill development. For example, you can modify kickball so that every child a chance to kick, run, and catch many times during the course of the game. Traditional kickball involves little activity and relatively little opportunity to develop basic skills. An alternative game divides the teams into pitchers and kickers. When a child is up, he or she either makes an out or a run. He must touch each base, but he doesn't have to follow a prescribed base path. As soon as one child kicks, another child in line is immediately up. Although the game looks unorganized, there is a tremendous amount of learning and practice going on.

Developing Basic Skills in Children

• Set aside regular times to work on the development of motor skills with children. Develop a structured plan. Introduce skills and systematically help them improve. Keeping a journal of the child's development will help you gradually introduce more difficult challenges. Conduct your movement and skill-development program in the spirit of fun and support. Encourage other children to join your home program.

• Encourage instruction in a variety of sports and movement experiences. Many gymnastics clubs and recreation departments have classes in movement exploration. Seek the maximum variety of exposure. Encourage participation in such activities as gymnastics, soccer, dancing, swimming, and running—activities that require children to move in ways. Although children need a certain amount of conditioning exercise, such as jogging and calisthenics, fitness is best developed through vigorous participation in sports and games.

• Encourage participation in organized athletics that emphasizes fundamentals and maximum participation. Organized sports are fine for children—so long as they don't overemphasize competition.

• Support and work for a good physical education program in the schools.

• Make physical fitness and sports an important part of family life. Children learn by example, and if their parents have a robust attitude toward life, they will usually conform to the family lifestyle.

• Provide understanding and support for "slower" children. Very often slow motor development is due to slower maturation. As these children mature, they will be perfectly capable of mastering movement skills. Immature children who are psychologically bruised may shun sports even when they do become developmentally mature.

Instant Replay

- Children grow rapidly during the first three years, less rapidly during childhood, then rapidly again at puberty. At any given age during childhood, girls are usually more mature than boys.

- Skill develops during childhood because of maturation and exposure to various movement experiences. Exposure to movement should be systematic—don't leave it to chance.

- Parents can stimulate children to move and develop perception during the earliest days of infancy.

- Children mature at different rates. Do not force children to progress too rapidly. Basic skills are important and are later integrated into more complex skills.

- Human contact is critical for the optimal development of perceptual and motor abilities.

- Encourage children and help them advance to more complex skills.

- Children learn best by doing and by imitating a good model. Don't intellectualize movement.

- Complex skills like throwing and catching can only be developed by practice. Avoid early competition for children if it means less practice in movement fundamentals.

- Don't over-structure exercise programs for children. Provide experiences for vigorous participation, maximum involvement, and fun.

- Support and work for a good elementary-school physical education program.

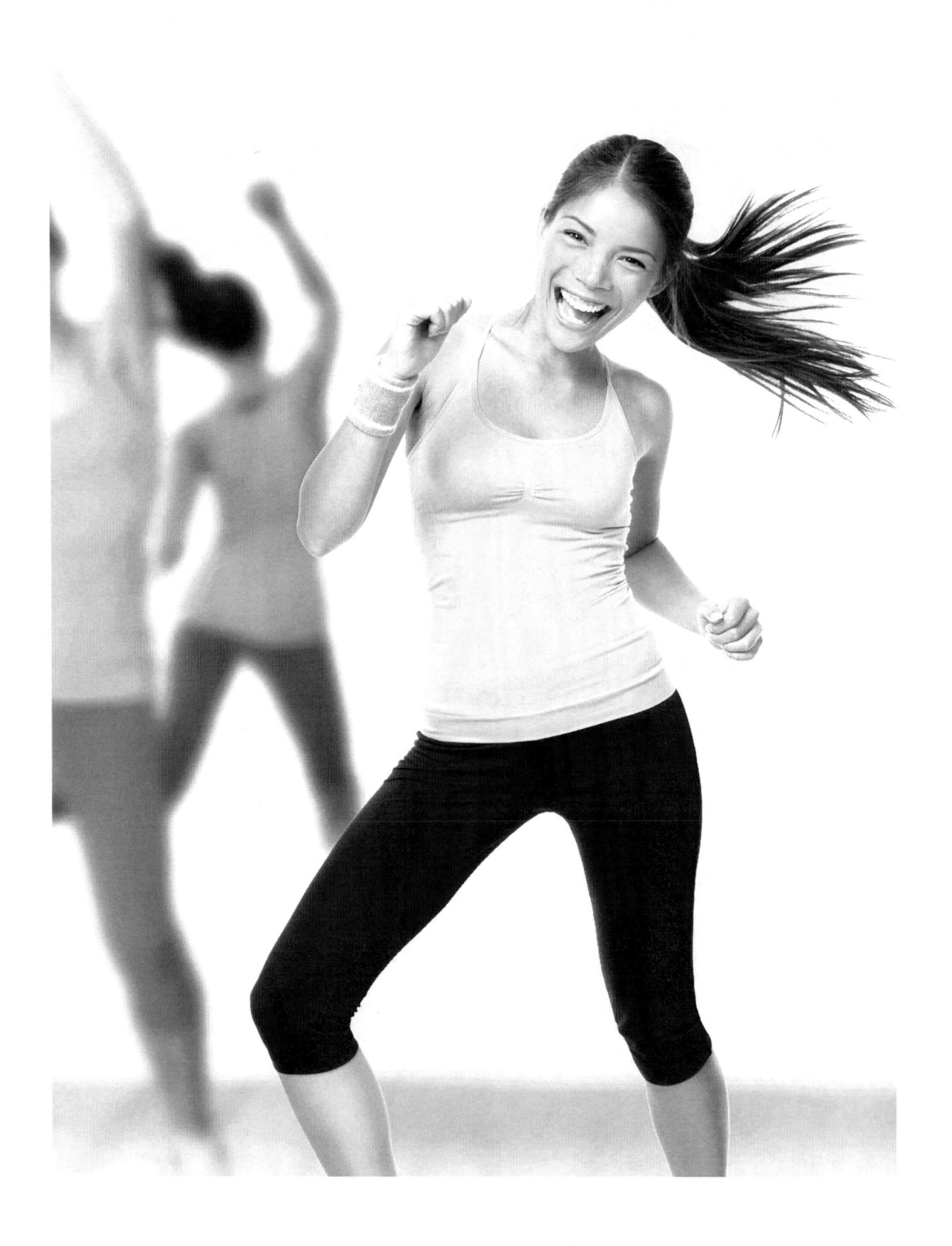

The Transition Years

PUBERTY & ADOLESCENCE

Bill is a twelve-year-old pitcher for the playground baseball team, and he's phenomenal, He can dazzle hitters with pitches that come across the plate blowing smoke. Bill looks more like a high school senior than a kid just out of elementary school. He dominates in all sports. He's better than the other kids-bigger, stronger, faster, and more agile. Most important, he is more physically mature. Is Bill destined for athletic stardom when he reaches high school and college? If he's this good as a twelve-year-old, won't he be a superstar when he's twenty?

It's extremely difficult to answer these questions. The prediction of physical performance from one age to another is guesswork at best. At any given age, fitness, skill, and athletic prowess are a product of genetics, maturation, and practice (or exposure). At puberty, maturationally advanced children may overshadow less mature children who may have the genetic potential to be superior when they're older. Yet the star athlete in junior high school is very often only average in high school or college.

Individual differences in maturation make it very difficult to predict athletic potential. Growth studies show that outstanding athletes in elementary school are usually not outstanding in junior high or high school. The exception to this is the top 1 to 2% of young athletes. Often, they are also top athletes when they are older.

Puberty and adolescence are difficult years for children. This is a period of emotional turbulence, and is a transition period when they go from the dependency of childhood to the independence of adulthood. Large differences in maturity can lead to feelings of insecurity in less developed children. Profound physical changestake place that cause anxiety and self-consciousness, even in physically advanced children.

Along with these physical and emotional changes comes a new capacity for learning motor skills. Children begin to develop the intellectual maturity to accept more structured sports and games and have increased attention spans. Pubescent child also have an increased ability to understand movement intellectually. You can place Less emphasis on informal play and movement exploration and concentrate more on skills and sports. Teen-aged children are more physically and emotionally prepared for more specialized competitive sports and more vigorous and structured training programs.

When children enter puberty, they do not become adults instantly. Puberty reflects a period of transition; you must understand these changes to help children become more skilled at sports and develop a love for physical activity.

The Body in Transition

The child's body changes dramatically during puberty and adolescence. There is no other period in life in which the body changes so substantially within such a short period of time. Emotionally, these changes can be difficult because they are experiencing a heightened sense of body awareness.

During adolescence, there is a rapid acceleration in the growth rate which coincides with the onset of sexual maturation—a period called puberty. This growth spurt is unique to humans and other primates, and all children experience it with its many predictable trials and tribulations. The growth spurt begins in girls between ten-and-a-half and thirteen and in boys between twelve-and-a-half and fifteen. The nature of the height gain depends on the age at which the growth spurt begins; late-maturing boys and girls tend to have longer legs and narrower hips than children who matured earlier. Early-maturing boys are often mesomorphs—characterized by stocky, muscular, and large-boned builds, while late-maturing boys tend to be ectomorphs, thinner and lankier than others. There are, of course, marked sex differences in physique at puberty. Boys are taller and have wider shoulders and more muscle, while girls have wider hips. Girls increase their subcutaneous fat (the layer of fat under the skin), while boys tend to lose theirs.

In girls, the adolescent growth spurt occurs at about the same time as the development of secondary sexual characteristics-the first sign of pubic hair and the beginning of breast development. The growth spurt is followed by the first menstrual period, a certain sign that puberty has begun. Physical exercise may affect the onset of menstruation and its regularity. Menarche, or the first menstruation, may not occur unless a girl has a certain percentage of fat in her body, takes in enough calories, and doesn't exercise excessively.

Girls begin increasing their body fat at about six years and continue at an increasing rate until about fifteen years of age. However, in some young female endurance athletes, such as swimmers and runners, vigorous training levels prevent the normal increase in fat and the onset of the menstrual periods is delayed. When the menstrual cycle does begin in these young women, it is often more irregular than in other girls. But when the level of vigorous training is reduced and the amount of body fat rises, the cycle usually becomes normal. The reasons for the effects of endurance exercise on menstrual periods are not known. One theory is that the body interprets low fat percentage as a kind of malnutrition, a condition not conducive to a normal pregnancy. Ammenorhea (lack of menstrual periods) can have serious, life-long effects. Even skipping one period can decrease bone density slightly. Years of irregular menstrual cycles can greatly increase fracture risks as a woman ages.

Boys have no single signal of puberty comparable to menarche; they develop adult levels of sperm production gradually. Pubic, axillary (armpit), and facial hair growth also takes place gradually. Yet the growth spurt in boys is much more pronounced than in girls; practically every muscle and body dimension is part of the accelerated growth during puberty.

The development of apocrine sweat glands cause anxiety in young teenagers. Apocrine sweat glands are located in the groin and armpit areas and in the feet; they are the glands that cause the legendary locker room odor. Sweat glands in the other parts of the body are called eccrine glands. Before puberty, the apocrine sweat glands remain inactive. Explain apocrine sweat gland growth to your child so that it doesn't become a problem.

Although muscle size increases in both sexes during puberty, boys develop bigger muscles because they have more testosterone. Sexually mature boys have about ten times more testosterone than girls. Testosterone produces the many male sexual characteristics; it causes boys to lose some of their "baby fat" and increases their capacity for muscle hypertrophy (enlargement) through training. At puberty, boys have a tremendous opportunity to gain muscle mass and strength rapidly. Weight training is effective for producing strength increases at this time because of testosterone triggers muscle growth. Weight training can be a great equalizer for a boy who was skinny or uncoordinated in the past. A vigorous weight training program at puberty causes physical improvement for any child, helps decrease body fat, and can lead to improved self-image and physical fitness. Other types of vigorous training, such as sprinting, interval training, and endurance training, are also more effective once testosterone levels increase. Although girls do not experience an increase in testosterone, they are capable of increasing their physical capacity because they become more physiologically mature.

Resting and maximum heart rates decrease in both girls and boys during puberty, but are greater in boys. Between fifteen and seventeen years, resting heart rate in boys is generally ten percent less than in girls, and maximum heart rate is about four beats per minute lower. Heart size and stroke volume (the amount of blood pumped per contraction of the heart) increase in both sexes, but the rise is more pronounced in boys. The capacity of the cardiovascular system is similar in boys and in girls during childhood, but a gap occurs at puberty and becomes greater and greater as adolescence progresses. Most of the difference in endurance capacity is due to sex differences in oxygen transport capacity. The hemoglobin count steadily increases in boys during early adolescence, which contributes to their endurance superiority because hemoglobin carries oxygen. More efficient chemical systems within muscles and an increased breathing capacity also contribute to rising endurance in boys during adolescence. Boys have more enzymes important in energy production, more and larger mitochondria (energy centers in cells), and a greater capacity to store glycogen, an important fuel for exercise. The higher breathing capacity in boys is due to their larger body size.

Systolic blood pressure—the maximum pressure in the arteries—rises during adolescence, but more in boys than in girls. Diastolic pressure—the minimum arterial pressure—remains the same for both sexes. Hypertension, or high blood pressure (high systolic and/or diastolic pressure), is a leading risk factor of coronary artery disease in adults. Children reach adult blood pressure values during the teen years, so it's important for blood pressure screening to begin at that time. The child should see a physician if you suspect high blood pressure.

Motor Development During Adolescence

Puberty and adolescence are periods of great motor development in boys and girls alike. The large increase in body size among boys is accompanied by a tremendous increase in the capacity to run, jump, throw, catch, balance, and move efficiently. Boys tend to continue improving in most movement skills until eighteen to twenty years of age.

Motor performance in girls levels off or declines during the teen years. Balancing ability remains the same, but running, jumping and throwing skills deteriorate. The increase in body fat and widening hips in girls may contribute. Women athletes typically achieve their highest levels of performance during their late teen years. Recent trends in athletics indicate that young women are capable of far greater levels of performance than was thought possible. Today's top women swimmers, for example, are equaling the performance levels of Olympic male swimmers of the early 1960s. Clearly, girls are capable of increasing their performance levels during adolescence. In the 2002 World Masters Games, 1972 swimming gold medal winner Shane Gould swam 2 seconds slower than her Olympic winning time, even though she was 45-years old. This suggests she could have swam much faster if she had stayed with the sport.

Social factors seem to be the primary reason for female performance characteristics during the teen years. Girls want to look attractive and don't want to attend class "all sweaty." Girls find it difficult to realize that physical fitness is in her best interest. The many benefits of sports and exercise for a teenage girl include:

• Contributing to a good figure by helping to control body fat. Thus, sports and exercise contribute to sex appeal.

• Contributing to a wellness lifestyle. Exercise is the most important health habit people can have to prevent heart disease and many types of cancer.

• Contributing to a positive self-image. A girl with a healthy, skillful body feels more self-assured and has more energy for the active teenage years.

• Contributing to the development of competitiveness, a trait essential to success in the business world. Today's women are much more likely to seek a career that will require the ability to compete. Sports teaches people to strive constantly to better themselves. During this process, self-confidence is developed because of the accomplishments that naturally occur.

Parents should take a special interest in your daughter's physical fitness. Let her know you consider exercise important. Try to involve her in family fitness activities and encourage interests that require physical fitness, such as skiing, camping, and hiking, tennis, and jogging. Don't preach-be a good example instead. These benefits apply, of course, to both boys and girls.

The positive effects of sports participation are not inevitable. Sports are not played in a vacuum. Some children are much more skilled than others, and slow learners may be ridiculed and made to feel very uncomfortable. An overweight child may be handicapped both socially and physically. Social problems can be so overwhelming that a positive outcome from sports may be difficult.

From Each According to His or Her Ability

A positive sports experience during adolescence doesn't happen by accident. I stressed this point in the chapter on infancy, and I stress it again here. Hopefully, the idea will be carried into adulthood. Children deserve individual programs consistent with their level of skill and natural abilities.

It's sad to see who won't participate in sports and physical activity because they're not good at it. The only way you can be good at a sport is to practice. Sure, some people catch on more quickly than others, but slow learners need more practice. Often a person will say, "I don't want to play-I'm no good at it." That person will never be good at it without some practice. A child who is deficient in sports skills should be encouraged to improve. The parent can take certain steps to maximize the development of sports skills and physical fitness:

• Stress the importance of an activity-oriented lifestyle. Make sure the child gets the opportunity to develop skills in recreation oriented lifetime sports and physical activities, such as jogging, tennis, racquetball, golf, horseback riding, swimming, and camping. Make sure you place emphasis on leisure time in addition to academics. Remember, overworked adults learned their habits as a child and teenager.

• Systematically work with the child to improve deficiencies in physical performance. For example, if the child has problems with throwing and catching, spend time working on these skills and encourage practice with other children. Encourage the child to learn new sports. (In Chapter 6 you will find some suggestions for helping children get started in lifetime sports.)

Help the child realize that it's a lot more fun to participate in sports than watching skilled professionals on the playing field. The new trend in participation was initially isolated to running. However, many people are discovering the joys of a well-rounded active lifestyle, and are clamoring to get on tennis courts, climbing wall, back country mountain trails, and ski slopes. Encourage this attitude of participation in children. With practice, they will have fun in a variety of activities.

Enjoyment of the active lifestyle requires a certain amount of skill. No one likes to appear uncoordinated. You can help your child develop skills and the self-confidence that goes with them through some systematic drill. It's not enough to play games alone. The child must develop well-rounded physical fitness. Emphasize endurance, strength, flexibility, speed, power, and skill. During adolescence, habits should be established that lead to a lifetime of well-rounded physical fitness. Children at this time can begin specific exercises to develop these physical fitness areas.

Developing Well-Rounded Physical Fitness

Physical fitness training is specific; heavy weight lifting may strengthen the shoulders, but it will do little or nothing to develop endurance. Likewise, sprinting on a track will not enhance shoulder flexibility or cardiovascular endurance. Children must work hard in each area of fitness to develop well-rounded physical fitness.

Developing Endurance

Endurance is one of the most important factors in a lifetime physical fitness program. Endurance training should become a regular part of a healthy lifestyle from the earliest school days—just as brushing your teeth, getting enough rest, and eating well. A healthy cardiovascular system plays an important part in reducing the risk of heart disease. You can live without an attractive body or a good cross-court backhand, but you can't live without a healthy heart and metabolism. Developing endurance fitness in teenagers will be easier if you understand some of the principles of endurance exercise:

• The best endurance exercises are those that use large muscle areas in a rhythmical manner for a long period of time. These exercises include walking, running, swimming, cycling, and cross-country skiing. Sports scientists have determined that endurance exercise should be practiced three to five days a week at at least 60 percent of maximum effort for 20 to 60 minutes if the goal is to improve fitness. At the very least, children should strive for at least 30 minutes a day of accumulated physical activity.

• To improve endurance, you must push your body harder than before. If you're running, for example, you must progressively run harder and faster than before if you want to improve.

Physical fitness is, to a great extent, a reflection of your activities. If you exercise a lot, you will be physically fit; if you don't, you will be out of shape. The harder you work, the better shape you'll be in. (There are hazards to overtraining, however. They are discussed in Chapter 5.)

• Start off gradually. If the child does too much too soon, his muscles will become sore and he might injure himself. Although it's important to push harder progressively, improvements should be made one step at a time. The keys to high levels of physical performance are consistency and regularity. The child must learn that to attain physical fitness, he must train for many years. As a child matures physically, he can train consistently over a long period of time; a high level of endurance fitness will become a reality. This is one reason why cardiovascular exercise is so good for teenagers.

• The endurance training program should be systematic, with a definite starting place and definite short-term goals for improvement.

- The intensity of an exercise can be determined by movement speed and heart rate.

The effects of exercise are extremely predictable for an individual child, however. The best way to assess these exercise effects is through a treadmill test, during which heart rate, oxygen consumption, and exercise capacity are monitored simultaneously. The treadmill test can determine two very important factors: the target heart rate and the ideal exercise training level. The target heart rate tells the exercise heart rate required for improvement; the ideal exercise training level tells how fast the child needs to run during training to improve his fitness. Target heart rate and ideal exercise training level actually provide the same information. You and your child can use one or both methods in designing the ideal program. Few children have a treadmill at their disposal, but there are other methods available to help adolescents determine the ideal exercise heart rate and exercise intensity.

The Target Heart Rate

Fitness is improved by exercising at high energy levels. Energy levels during exercise can be estimated by measuring the heart rate.

The maximal heart rate is the fastest level at which the heart can beat. The target heart rate is between 70 and 85 percent of the maximal heart rate. The target heart rate tells the best possible level at which to exercise. It is really a measure of the minimum level of exercise you must do in order to improve fitness.

Measuring Maximal Heart Rate

Maximal heart rate is usually measured on a treadmill. A person works at an exhaustive level of exercise, and the highest heart rate recorded is the maximal heart rate. There are other methods, however, of estimating the maximal heart rate without a treadmill:

- Maximal heart rate is related to age. As a rule of thumb, maximal heart rate is equal to 220 minus the person's age. A fifteen-year-old would be expected to have a maximum heart rate of 205 beats per minute (220 - 15 = 205). However, maximal heart rates in teenagers are extremely variable, ranging from about 180 beats per minute to almost 230. For many children then, this simple method is inappropriate and inaccurate.

- Estimate maximal heart rate by measuring the heart rate after a one-minute all-out sprint. Have the child run 300 to 500 yards as fast as possible. Then measure the heart rate for ten seconds immediately after the sprint. Multiply this ten-second heart rate by six to get the maximal one-minute heart rate. It's very important to get the heart rate during the first ten seconds; any delay will result in an underestimating of the maximum.

A word of caution: an all-out sprint should be conducted with great care. The child should warm up thoroughly by walking, running, and stretching. This test should not be attempted until the child has been running regularly for at least four weeks. I do not recommend this test for adults unless they are physically fit.

Determining the Target Heart Rate from the Maximal Heart Rate

Step 1. Determine the maximal heart rate.
Step 2. Look up the target heart rate on the following chart.

Maximal Heart Rate	Target Heart Rate
220	175
218	174
216	172
214	171
212	169
210	168
208	167
206	165
204	164
202	162
200	161
198	160
196	158
194	157
192	155
190	154
188	153
186	151
184	150
182	148
180	147

Using the Target Heart Rate

You can use the target heart rate to determine the proper level of intensity at which to exercise. The heart rate during the first ten minutes of recovery from exercise is the same as the heart rate during exercise. You can compare your exercise heart rate with the target heart rate to determine if you're working hard enough.

In order to measure the exercise heart rate, you will need a stopwatch or a watch with a second hand. Teach the child how to measure the pulse either at the wrist or by placing a hand directly over the heart.

The procedures for measuring exercise heart rate are:

1. Take the pulse for ten seconds immediately after exercise. Multiply this value by six to get

the exercise pulse rate. It's easier for the child to remember the ten-second equivalent for the target heart rate rather than the full-minute count. For example, an exercise heart rate of 150 derives from a ten-second count of 25 (25 x 6 = 150).

2. Have the child compare the exercise heart rate with the target heart rate. If the exercise heart rate is not high enough, then he or she is not working hard enough.

The target heart rate is a built-in speedometer. If the child knows the target heart rate, he will always know if he's getting a good workout. As he gets in better shape and his pulse drops at a particular speed, the target heart rate tells him that he must go faster to benefit from training.

This procedure may be confusing at first, but it's worth the trouble. Remember, high levels of fitness are attained only by systematically increasing the intensity of exercise. The heart rate is a built-in indicator of when to run faster. If you establish the habit of measuring heart rate when your child is young, he or she will get the most out of exercise.

Short-Term Running Goals

Improvement in running is easiest when the child has a series of goals to shoot for. These goals are easy to calculate-all the child needs to know is the correct starting point.

An ideal running program does not require the child to run at full speed all the time. The best running program requires the child to run at about 70 to 85 percent of maximum. To run at this level, the child needs to know his or her maximum capacity. I have prepared a chart to help teenagers determine their maximum capacity and set up an appropriate running program. The test requires the child to run one and a half miles as fast as possible; running time is then used to determine the proper running goals.

1.5-Mile Run Test

The 1 1/2-mile run test should be preceded by at least four weeks of running. If a child isn't used to running long distances, he or she should follow the suggested four-week preliminary conditioning program and take the 1.5-mile test at the end of the fourth week.

Week	Workout	Days per Week
Week 1	Run and walk 1 mile	5
Week 2	Run and walk 1.5 miles	5
Week 3	Run 1 mile and walk 1 mile	5
Week 4	Run 1.5 miles and walk 1 mile	5

If the child has any medical problems, such as heart or lung problems, diabetes, or obesity, have him see a doctor before he takes the test or begins the pre-test conditioning program. Instructions for the 1.5-mile test:

1. Take this test on a 440-yard (1/4-mile) track. Most high schools and colleges have this distance track. Use a stopwatch or a watch with a second hand to time the run.

2. Have the child warm up by running, walking, and stretching. Don't, however, let. him warm up so much that he becomes fatigued.

3. Tell the child to run the one and a half miles as fast as possible. If he gets tired, tell him to walk, but to keep moving.

4. Refer to the 1.5-Mile Run Test Chart (below) to determine the appropriate starting place in the Running Program Chart. For example, if a child ran the one and a half miles in 12:01, he would start at step 22 in the running program.

1.5-Mile Run Test

Time (min:sec)	Starting Step of Running Program
8:55	33
9:10	32
9:31	30
9:50	29
10:16	28
10:35	26
11:01	25
11:31	23
12:01	22
12:35	20
13:10	18
13:50	16
14:31	15
15:20	13
16:10	10
17:16	8
18:25	6
19:40	4
21:16	1

The Running Program

The running program provides the teenager with a series of short-term goals. This program will produce gradual increases in endurance capacity and produce incentives for improvement.

- The child enters at a particular step determined by his performance on the 1.5-mile run test, and will not usually begin at step 1. The faster the time on the 1.5-mile test, the higher the starting step.

- The child remains at a step until it begins to feel easier to run at that speed. Remember, the step should not require maximum effort. The child can use his or her heart rate to help determine if it's time to increase a step.

Running, of course, is not the only kind of endurance exercise that will develop the cardiovascular system. Running does, however, produce the greatest training effects in the shortest period of time. Teenagers should use running as their primary means of conditioning. Although swimming and cycling also produce cardiovascular endurance, they usually don't prove vigorous enough when practiced at a noncompetitive level. Cycling and swimming are highly recommended as part of the program, but only as supplements to running.

Running Program

Step	Distance (Miles)	Target Time	Time per Mile
1	1.5	24:31	16:21
2	1.5	23:55	15:57
3	1.5	23:20	15:34
4	1.5	22:46	15:11
5	1.5	22:13	14:49
6	1.5	21:40	14:27
7	1.5	21:09	14:06
8	1.5	20:38	13:45
9	1.5	20:08	13:25
10	2.0	26:11	13:05
11	2.0	25:33	12:46
12	2.0	24:55	12:28
13	2.0	24:19	12:09
14	2.0	23:43	11:52
15	2.0	23:08	11:34
16	2.0	22:35	11:17
17	2.0	22:02	11:01

Continued on next page.

Step	Distance (Miles)	Target Time	Time per Mile
18	2.0	21:29	10:45
19	2.0	20:58	10:29
20	2.0	20:27	10:14
21	2.5	24:57	9:59
22	2.5	24:20	9:44
23	2.5	23:44	9:30
24	2.5	23:10	9:16
25	2.5	22:36	9:02
26	2.5	22:03	8:49
27	2.5	21:30	8:36
28	2.5	20:59	8:24
29	2.5	20:28	8:11
30	3.0	23:58	7:59
31	3.0	23:23	7:48
32	3.0	22:49	7:36
33	3.0	22:15	7:25
34	3.0	21:43	7:14
35	3.0	21:11	7:04
36	3.0	20:40	6:53
37	3.0	20:10	6:43
38	3.5	22:57	6:33
39	3.5	22:23	6:24
40	3.5	21:51	6:14
41	3.5	21:19	6:05
42	3.5	20:47	5:56
43	3.5	20:17	5:48
44	4.0	22:37	5:39
45	4.0	22:04	5:31
46	4.0	21:32	5:23
47	4.0	21:00	5:15
48	4.0	20:29	5:07
49	4.5	22:29	4:60
50	4.5	21:56	4:53

Developing Speed and Agility

Systematic development of speed should begin during adolescence. Speed is improved by participating in start-and-stop sports, such as basketball, soccer, tennis, racquetball, and field hockey. However, this is not enough. Running fast falls under the same training rules as other aspects of fitness: You can't run fast without regular practice and systematic increases in running speed.

Speed is important for enjoyment and success in many sports. There are many aspects of speed: running fast, rapidly changing direction, maintaining balance in difficult circumstances, and stopping and starting rapidly. In most sports, a person not only has to run fast, but run fast repeatedly. In tennis, for example, if you lose your speed and agility to fatigue after the first couple of sets, you will probably lose the match. There are a variety of exercise techniques to improve speed and agility; these include interval training, plyometrics, weight training, agility drills, and rope skipping. Repeated practice of these exercises will not only develop speed and agility, but will improve the specific speed endurance and power needed in sports.

Interval Training

Interval training—repeated bouts of high-intensity exercise—has been popular since the late 1950s. Interval training develops speed and the fitness necessary for start-and-stop sports. There are many possible types of interval training, each with a different training result. For example, the football or tennis player will train to run very short distances very fast, since this is what those games require. The miler would practice running faster over a longer period of time. The marathon runner would engage in long-distance interval training.

Interval training is an important method that can help any child reach high levels of fitness. It consists of four components: distance, speed, repetitions, and rest intervals between repetitions.

Physically, interval training is very demanding. It has two possible pitfalls: injury and overtraining. These possibilities can be minimized by thorough warm-up and limiting interval practice to 2-3 days a week.

Following are three interval running programs that you can adapt to fit the child's needs exactly:

Short-Sprint Intervals

Short-sprint intervals are sometimes called wind-sprints.

- **Distance**: The distance can vary between 5 and about 220 yards. Short distances of under 40 yards develop the ability to start rapidly, vital to success in many sports. Longer short-sprint intervals of 220 yards develop endurance for high-intensity exercise, but are less valuable for developing maximum speed over a short distance.

- **Speed**: The speed in short-sprint intervals should always be 90 to 100 percent of maximum. These intervals specifically provide the opportunity to use high-speed muscle fibers. Anything less than maximum effort is virtually useless.

THE TRANSITION YEARS

- **Repetitions:** As a rule of thumb, the greater the number of repetitions, the slower each individual repetition should be. If the goal is to develop speed, then too many repetitions will be inappropriate. The number of repetitions is also determined by the child's fitness level. If the interval distance is 40 yards and the child is in great shape, then 20 repetitions may be acceptable. However, if the child has just started serious training, then even four or five repetitions may be too many.

- **Rest Interval between Repetitions:** The rest interval is determined by the physical fitness of the child. The rest interval for 60 yards may be less than 30 seconds while the rest interval for 220 yards may be up to five or six minutes. If there is insufficient rest time, speed will decrease. In general, rest until breathing begins to return to normal.

Example of short-sprint interval training:
Distance: 50 yards
Speed: 6.5 seconds
(90 percent of maximum)
Repetitions: 5
Rest between
repetitions: 2 minutes

Middle-Distance Intervals

This training is beneficial for developing fitness for high-intensity sports and for developing the ability to sustain speed in middle-distance running (400 yards to one mile).

- **Distance:** Middle distances range from 220 to 800 yards. The longer the distance, the greater the involvement and importance of the heart and lungs.

- **Speed:** Speed ranges from 60 to 100 percent of maximum, depending on the fitness level of the child, the number of interval repetitions, and the rest between repetitions. This training is excellent for improving the ability to run faster for a longer period of time.

- **Repetitions:** Repetitions depend upon the other factors of interval training. For example, running even one full-effort 440 can be extremely difficult. Top endurance athletes, however, can run up to twenty 440s in less than 65 seconds each.

- **Rest Intervals:** Rest intervals can vary from five minutes of complete rest to a slow jog (220 to 440 yards) between repetitions.

Example of middle-distance interval training:
Distance: 440 yards
Speed: 80 seconds
Repetitions: 4
Rest between
repetitions: 5 minutes

Long-Distance Intervals

Long-distance intervals increase the child's ability to run faster over greater distances. For example, if a child's goal is to run three miles in 24 minutes (three eight-minute miles), he or she may practice repeatedly running one-mile runs in seven minutes and 45 seconds.

- **Distance:** 800 yards to six miles. Longer distances do little for speed development, but can aid the development of a faster running pace over long distances.

- **Speed:** Longer intervals are generally used to run at the desired pace of a long distance run over a shorter distance, so the speed should either be at or slightly faster than the desired pace of the run.

- **Repetitions**: Longer intervals make too many repetitions difficult.

- **Rest Intervals**: Rest intervals can range from five or ten minutes to all day. A six-mile interval, for example, might be run in the morning and in the afternoon.

Jumping Rope

Jumping rope is a very intricate skill that requires the coordination of visual perception with simultaneous movements of the arms and legs. Encourage the child to learn these intricate hand and foot movements, and to turn the rope at faster speeds. The best jump rope is made of leather and has wood handles that contain bearings, which make the rope turn more easily and prevent tangles.

Jumping rope can be used as a cardiovascular exercise. Jumping rope for 1-5 minutes will develop endurance fitness quickly because of its high intensity can be practiced as interval training. For example, the child could alternate between jumping for one minute and resting for one minute.

Agility Exercise

Agility is the ability to integrate basic movement skills into sports movements. During childhood, emphasis should be placed upon basic movement skills. During adolescence, these basic skills should be incorporated into a variety of more complex skills. The agile person is one who can use basic movement skills in novel ways under a variety of circumstances. You can improve agility by working on exercises that require a synthesis of primary movement skills.

Agility Drills

Agility drills can be conducted like interval training. In fact, you can substitute some of these drills for short-sprint intervals.

- **Slant Running.** Have the child run straight for a few steps, then at an angle, either to the left or right. Many variations of this exercise can be used: the child could add forward rolls on the grass, 360-degree turns during the run, or abrupt starts and stops.

- **Backward Running.** Begin by running backward slowly. Gradually, the child should increase his speed to a sprint. Slant running can also be incorporated into this exercise.

- **Hurdles.** Run and jump over hurdles or low benches placed either in sequence or in an obstacle course.

- **Figure Eights.** Run in figure-eight patterns. As skill increases, make the figure eights smaller. This develops the ability to change directions rapidly.

Speed Exercises

Children are born with a certain speed potential. All the training in the world isn't going to make the slow kid break the world record in the 100-meter dash. However, any child can become faster and better conditioned. Practice makes the difference. The kid who works hard consistently will eventually leave the others in the dust. These are only a few of the many speed and agility exercises possible.

Developing Flexibility

Unfortunately, the great flexibility of the infant is often lost during childhood. Make sure that stretching is a regular part of your child's exercise routine. Vigorous sports may result in injury if the child doesn't have good joint mobility. Make sure your child understands the basic principles of stretching:

• Flexibility should be increased gradually. Too much stretching exercise all at once is an open invitation to injury.

• Stretch after exercise when the muscles are warm. There is no evidence that pre-exercise stretching prevents injury.

• To perform flexibility exercises properly, stretch until you feel a perceptible pull in the muscles. Try to hold that position for 15 to 30 seconds. Relax for a moment and then repeat the stretch.

• Flexibility exercises can provide many benefits. Some but not all evidence suggests that post-workout stretching will reduce post-exercise muscle soreness.

• A fuller range of motion in joints can only be gained through consistent, regular exercise. You've got to work systematically toward increasing flexibility.

• Never bounce during stretching exercises. Bouncing can result in pulls and tears in muscles, and can activate the body's stretch receptors, which may cause muscle cramps that are sometimes severe.

• Never overstretch. Do not try to stretch beyond the threshold of pain. With practice and patience, you will eventually be able to exceed this point in your flexibility exercises.

There are hundreds of flexibility exercises. Following are some of the basic movements. Encourage your child to develop flexibility in many joints. Here are exercises for many parts of the body:

Alternate Leg Stretcher

This exercise stretches the hamstrings, hip, knee, ankle, and buttocks. Lie on your back with both legs straight. (a) Grasp your left leg behind the thigh, and pull in to your chest. (b) Hold this position, then extend your left leg toward the ceiling. (c) Hold this position, then bring your left knee back to your chest and pull your toes toward your shin with your left hand. Stretch the back of the leg by attempting to straighten your knee. Repeat for the other leg.

Sitting Stretches

Sit on the floor, legs outstretched, with your feet about six inches apart. Slowly reach toward your foot and grab your leg as far down as possible, moving your head as close to your knee as you can. Hold the stretch for 20 to 30 seconds. Relax and then repeat, alternating between left and right. Sitting stretches are excellent for the back and hamstring muscles.

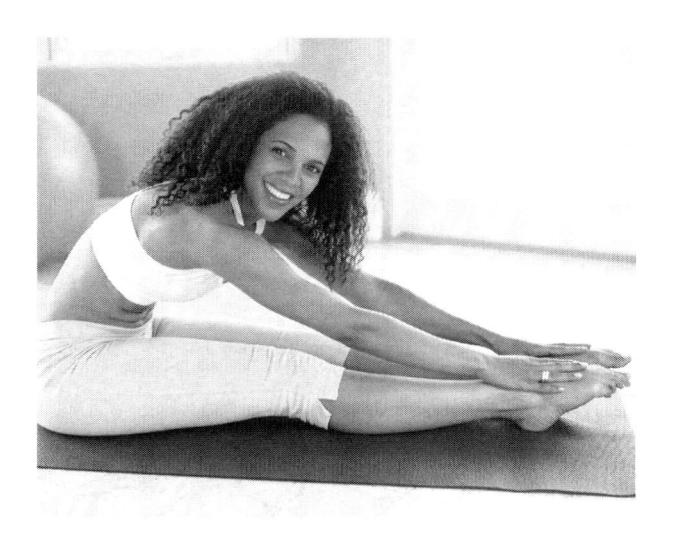

Sitting Stretches

Back Rolls

Sit on the floor with your legs bent and your feet flat. Pull your knees toward your chest and gently roll backward. Hold that position for 30 seconds. Relax a moment, then repeat.

Groin Stretches

The groin is particularly susceptible to injury in high-intensity sports like tennis and basketball. A good stretch before the game, though, can ward off injury and prepare the muscles for action. Sit on the floor and put the soles of your feet together. Then gently press the inside of your knees with your elbows until you feel a noticeable pull in the groin area. Hold this position for 20 to 30 seconds, relax a moment, and then repeat.

Step Stretch

This exercise stretches the hip and the muscles on the front of the thigh (quadriceps). From a standing position, step forward and flex your forward knee, keeping your knee directly above your ankle. Stretch your other leg back so that it is parallel to the floor. Press your hips forward and down to stretch. Your arms can be at your sides.l, on top of your knee, or on the ground for balance. Repeat on on the other side.

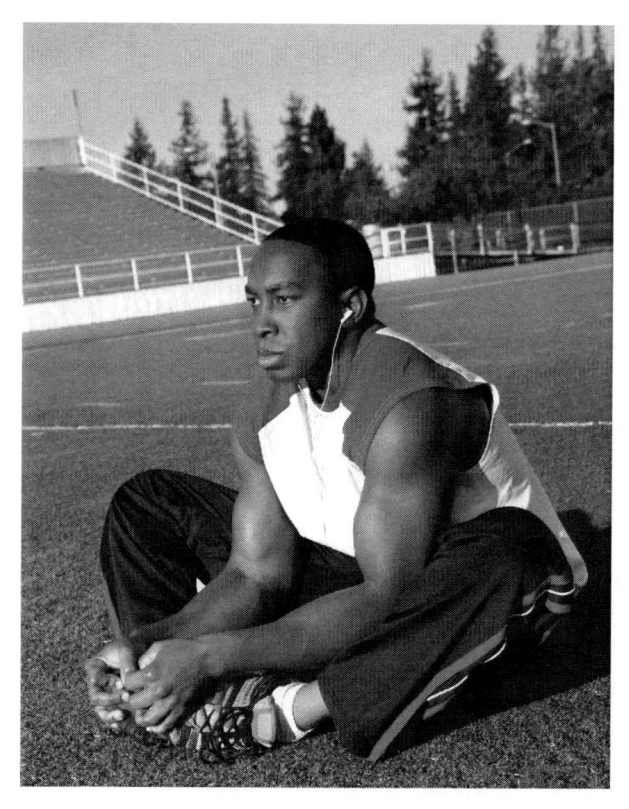

Groin Stretches

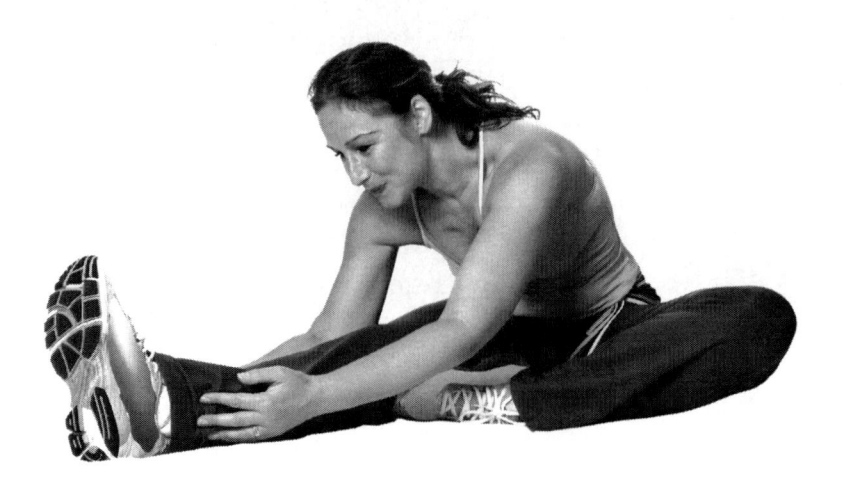

Hurdler Stretch: Hamstrings

Modified Hurdler Stretches: Hamstrings (back thigh muscles)

From the modified hurdler position—sitting, one leg extended and the other foot placed on the inner thigh of the extended leg—bend forward until you feel muscle tension in the back of your leg. Relax and repeat, and then alternate positions to perform the stretch on the other leg.

Shoulder Hangs

Find a chin-up bar that is high enough off the ground to dangle freely from. Simply hang for 10 to 30 seconds.

Hip Stretches

With your feet about eighteen inches from a wall, archway, or lamp post, lean against the surface with your hand or forearm and thrust your hip inward. Keep that position for 20 to 30 seconds, then relax and repeat. Change sides and perform the exercise with the other hip. Joggers find this exercise especially valuable because it can prevent the hip soreness that often results from running.

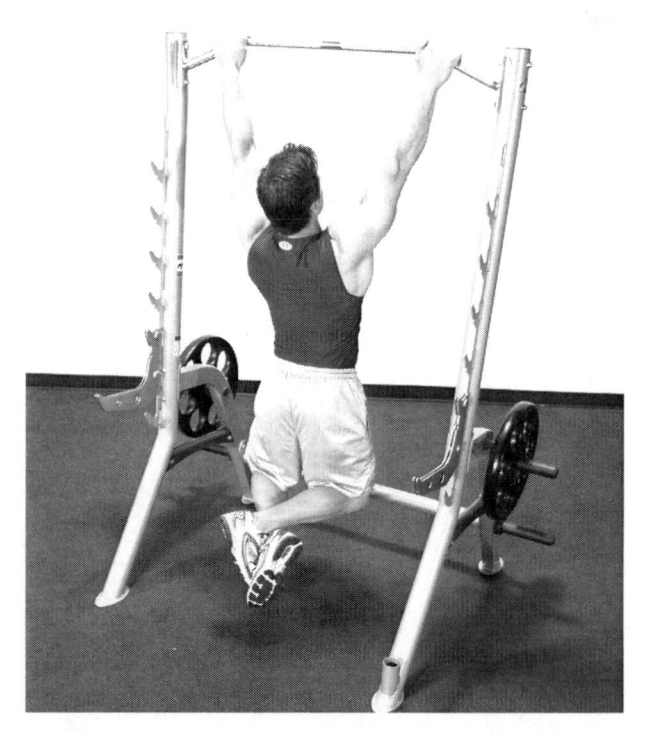

Shoulder Hang

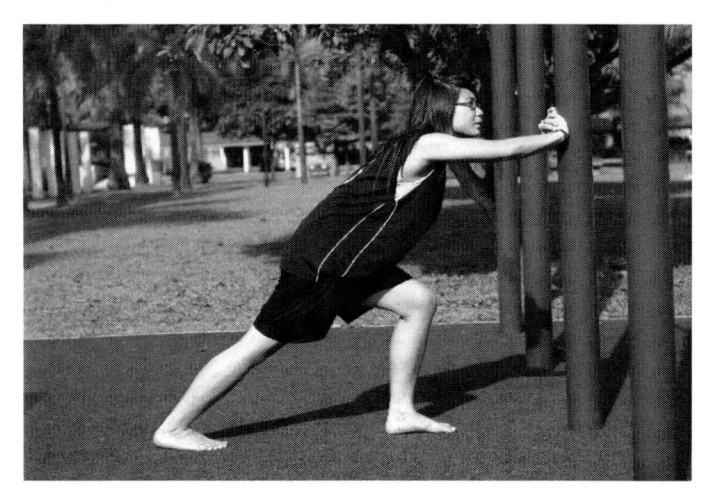

Achilles Tendon Stretch

Shoulder Circles with a Towel

Grip a towel at both ends, keeping your hands slightly farther than shoulder-width apart. Slowly bring your hands over your head and continue going backward until you're holding the towel behind your back. Shoulder circles are great for increasing flexibility. As you become more supple, perform the exercise holding your hands closer together.

Achilles Tendon Stretches

Stand a few feet away from a wall. Without moving your legs, lean against the wall. You will feel a pull in your Achilles tendon and in your calf muscles. Hold the position for a moment or two, return, and repeat. This exercise can also be performed by stretching one leg at a time. Achilles tendon stretches are invaluable to runners.

Shin Stretches

Assume a kneeling position, with the tops of your feet pressed against the floor. Gently sit back on your heels until you feel a stretch in your shins and in the top part of your foot. These exercises are valuable in preventing shin splints, which commonly afflict Joggers.

Footsies

With your leg outstretched, rotate your foot through its entire range of motion: flex and extend your toes and twist your foot inward and outward. Then do the exercise with the other foot. Footsies are great if your feet are sore in the morning. Try doing them before you get out of bed.

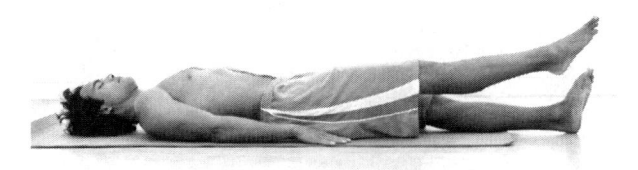

Footsies

THE TRANSITION YEARS

Developing Strength

Strength exercises are important for teenage boys and girls alike. Muscle strength can be developed with the body weight used as resistance, with weights, or with exercise machines. Muscle strength is an important attribute in most sports, providing a valuable reserve for endurance sports, power for sports like tennis, basketball, and baseball, and helping to prevent injury in sports like football.

Strength training is both physically and emotionally valuable to the child. A less-skilled or late-maturing child may be able to close the gap on his peers by beginning vigorous strength training during puberty.

Strength Training without Equipment

Because of gravity, our bodies are a kind of built-in gymnasium. To lift the body weight against gravity requires a lot of muscle power, but every child should be able to handle his or her own body weight. The following exercises, although not as good as weight training for developing strength, have an advantage, as they can be done anywhere without equipment. They use the body weight as resistance. Have your child try to do all of the sets suggested before moving on to a new exercise.

Leg Exercises

Phantom Chair (wall sits)

Skiers frequently use this exercise to develop greater flexibility and increase muscle strength in the legs. Keeping your feet flat on the floor, press your back up against a wall and align your thighs parallel with the floor-as if you were sitting in a straight-backed chair. Extend your arms in front of you, palms downward. At first, hold this position for 15 to 30 seconds. Gradually increase the time until you can "sit" in the phantom chair for three minutes. When you reach that level of endurance, try to do three repetitions.

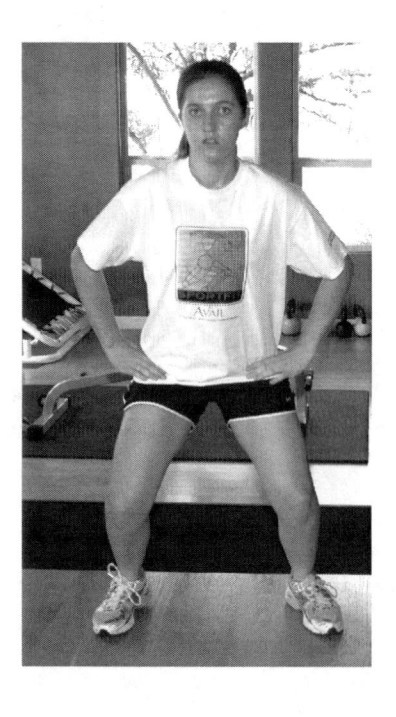

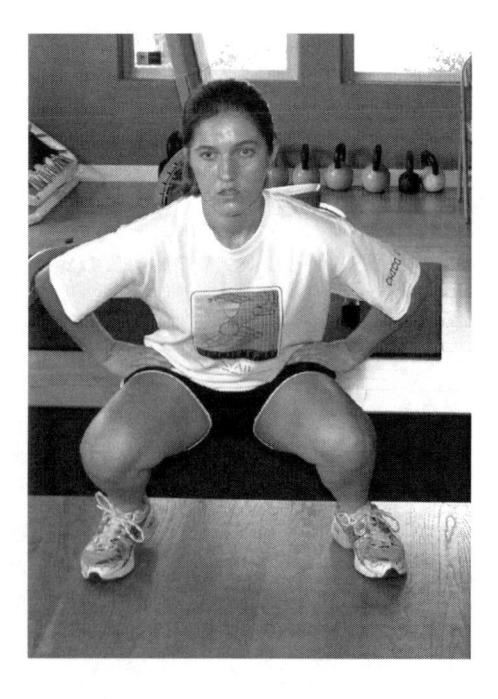

Knee Bends

Knee Bends

Place your feet about shoulder-width apart and bend your knees until your thighs are parallel to the floor. Complete three sets of 10 repetitions each. As your flexibility increases, vary the exercise by doing the knee bends more slowly. Go down gradually to a count of five, then return slowly to the standing position.

Step-Ups

Simply step up on a bench or chair. Do three sets, each consisting of 10 repetitions with the left leg and 10 with the right.

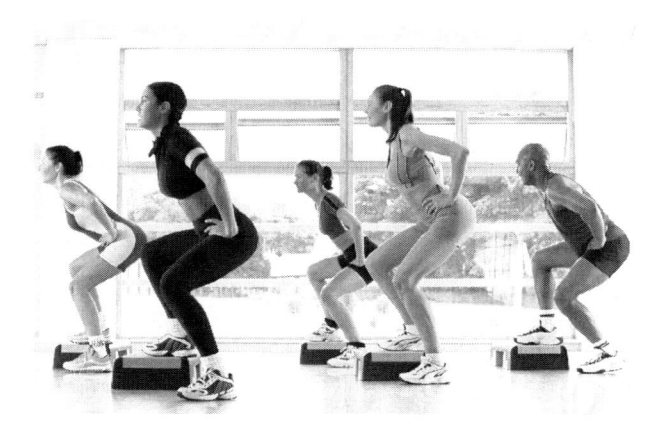

Step-Ups (here done with platforms)

Stair Climbing

This exercise can be done on any staircase that has more than five steps. A football stadium is the ideal place. Begin by running up 10 to 20 stairs, and gradually increase both the number and the intensity. A word of caution: Don't overdo this exercise. Start out easy and build up at a moderate pace.

Heel Raises

Stand upright and simply lift your heels off the floor, so that your weight is on the balls of your feet and your toes. Slowly return to standing position. You'll feel this exercise strengthening your thighs and calves. Do three sets of 10 to 20 repetitions each.

Stomach Exercises

Bent-Knee Sit-Ups

Lie on your back, place your feet flat on the floor, and bend your knees. Clasp your hands behind your head, and bring your elbows to your knees. If this type of sit-up is too difficult, try the same motion with your arms folded across your chest rather than with your hands behind your head. Either way, remember to keep your knees bent. This will prevent back strain and exercise your stomach muscles more thoroughly than straight-leg sit-ups. Begin with 10 sit-ups, and gradually build up to two or three sets of 50 repetitions each.

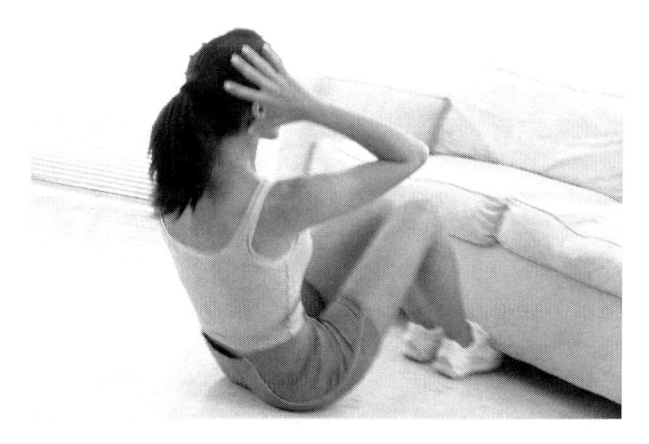

Bent-Knee Sit-Ups

Side Bends

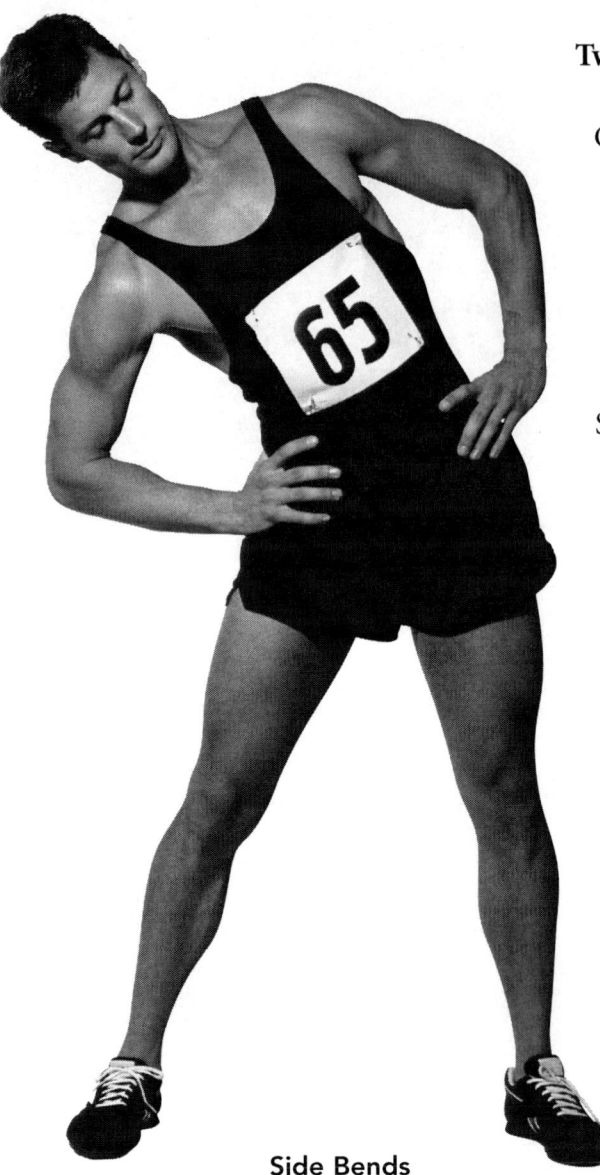

Twists

Grip a broom handle with both hands, resting it on your shoulders behind your neck. Simply rotate from left to right and right to left. Complete three sets of 25 to 50 repetitions each.

Side Bends

Stand erect with your arms at your sides. Bend to one side and then the other, keeping your knees straight. Do three sets of 25 to 50.

Upper Body Exercises

Chin-Ups (pull-ups)

Use a chin-up bar in a schoolyard, or purchase one that will fit in a doorway. Grip the bar, palms facing whichever way is most comfortable, and try to pull yourself up. Most people have a lot of trouble with this exercise. If you can't pull yourself all the way up, simply hang from the bar for 10 seconds three times. Even this will increase your strength. With practice, you will eventually be able to pull yourself all the way up. When you can, build up to three sets of 10 chin-ups each.

Push-Ups

Lie on the floor in a prone position, supporting yourself on your hands and toes. Keeping your body straight, push yourself up off the floor and then lower yourself down again. Be sure to keep your back straight and your stomach firm during the exercise. If you have difficulty at first, modify the push-up by supporting yourself on your knees instead of your toes. Build up to three sets of 20 push-ups each.

Parallel Bar Dips

You can find dip bars in many schoolyards and college and high school gyms. With your arms straight, begin by supporting yourself between the bars. Lower yourself between the bars, then push up to the starting position. Begin with 1 to 5 repetitions; gradually increase to three sets of 10 repetitions.

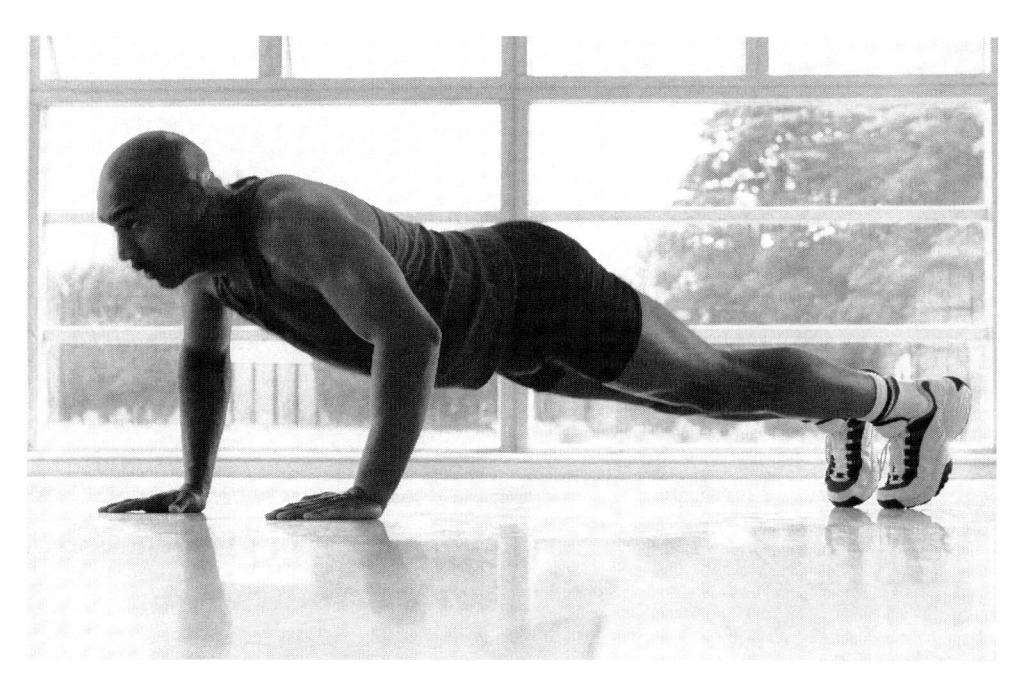

Push-Ups

Weight Training

Weight training is the best type of exercise for developing strength for sports. It is recommended for both boys and girls after they have reached puberty. Many studies suggest that pre-pubertal children can train with weights. Most children don't have the discipline to benefit from weight training before the teen years. As with other types of exercise, maximum benefit is only realized with consistent training over a long period of time.

You can get your child started with weight training by setting up a home gym. You can purchase weights at a sports store, but shop around before you buy-a 100-pound barbell set can vary in cost by as much as $30 at different stores. Weight sets with plastic plates can be so large that it's difficult to put much weight on the bar. Look around until you find equipment that suits the space in your home and your child's needs. Buy a weight set that allows for increases in strength.

Most children will be very surprised at how much weight they are capable of lifting. Many high school boys bench press well over 300 pounds. A high level of strength is a tremendous advantage in many sports. For example, weight training has contributed to the high performance levels in women's swimming. To develop a high level of strength in the home gym, provide your child with good equipment and stress the importance of safety.

Components of the Home Gymnasium

- **Barbell Set**. For the beginner, a 125-pound barbell set will be sufficient. However, there should be room on the bar for additional plates to be added as the child increases his or her strength. For the more advanced child, an Olympic-type weight lifting bar may be appropriate. The Olympic-type set allows the use of more weight and is easier to balance.

- **Adjustable Dumbbells.** These are not absolutely essential, but they allow the child to perform a greater variety of strength exercises.

- **Bench with Supports.** Buy or make a sturdy, padded bench. The weight supports should be strong enough to hold 500 to 600 pounds without toppling over onto the bench. The supports can either stand independently or be connected directly to the bench. Inquire at a gymnasium supply company for a bench that will fit your needs.

- **Squat Racks.** Squat racks must be sturdy or a serious injury may result. They should be adjusted to the height of the child.

- **Optional Equipment.** There are countless weight training contraptions available for the home gym. These include curl bars, dip bars, pull-up bars, incline and decline benches, lat machines, curl benches, power racks, lifting platforms, and pulleys. These devices can be purchased through gymnasium supply companies. Check the advertising in weight lifting magazines.

Safety in the Home Gymnasium

Safety should be your biggest concern when you set up a home gym. Follow the rules of weight room safety:

- Buy the best possible equipment you can afford. Inexpensive equipment may not be strong enough and may therefore be unsafe.

- Never allow your child to exercise alone. Make sure there is always a spotter present to give assistance when needed. Make sure the spotter understands the duties involved. There are an average of five deaths per year in home gyms in the United States. Most occur when children and teens lift without spotters.

- Never allow horseplay in the weight room.

- Be sure the child understands the importance of the warm-up in preventing injury.

- Be sure the weights are firmly fastened to the bar with collars.

Joining a Gymnasium or Health Club

The best way for a high school student to develop high levels of strength is to join a health club or gym. Teenagers can train at the high school, YMCA, or recreation center very inexpensively. Many health clubs offer student discounts. Public gyms usually have better equipment than most people can afford and provide a better, safer environment for strength training. Find out where the older kids are training before you run to the nearest health club (experienced athletes usually find the best places to train). Start off with an introductory membership of six weeks or so. Don't let them sign your child up for long-term contracts.

Principles of Weight Training

Weight training can be hard, boring work. It's important that your child get the maximum benefit from the training session by following these principles of weight training:

- Remember the "overload principle": each workout should be just a little harder than the last one. Don't expect to improve without consistently making new gains.

- Begin with one set of 8-10 repetitions for 8-10 exercises. Have the child do more sets as he or she gets stronger and is willing to devote more time to the program.

- Your ability to exert a lot of force all at once can be improved by doing fewer repetitions (1 to 5) with more weight.

- In general, weight lifters do many repetitions of an exercise in each set, and then many sets. Top bodybuilders spend as many as six hours a day in the training gym.

- Girls will usually not develop large muscles from weight training. Muscles need high levels of testosterone to grow substantially. Girls will lose fat through weight training, though, and develop a considerable amount of the strength that's required for sports. Don't let your daughter overlook this important component of fitness.

- It's best to train with weights three times per week. Any more than that can result in overtraining and little or no muscle gain. Pick specific days of the week, such as Monday, Wednesday, and Friday, and stick to them. Two days per week is the minimum amount of time you can spend on weight training and still benefit from it.

- Always perform your large-muscle exercises first. Your smaller muscles will fatigue more quickly than your larger ones, and limit your ability to complete and gain from the large-muscle exercises. For example, fatigued wrists or biceps that cannot carry their load during shoulder and chest exercises will limit the strength gains in those large muscles.

- Do your workout as quickly and efficiently as you can. Don't let yourself be distracted by gym chatter; you won't get any work done. Hustle! Unless you're heavily involved in strength training, your workout should not exceed an hour and a half.

- Always warm up before doing a set of full-strength large-muscle exercises, such as bench presses, squats, etc. Perform the exercise with less weight before you really go for it.

Basic Weight Training Exercises

When beginning a weight training program, have your child select a weight for each exercise that will allow him or her to do ten repetitions comfortably. For the first workout your child should do only one set of each exercise. Then gradually increase to three sets (this usually takes four to six workouts). There are countless exercises and numerous program variations. I've put together some good basic exercises an adolescent can do with a barbell set at home:

Squats

Rest a barbell on your shoulders behind your neck, keeping your legs a comfortable distance apart. You might try putting a one-inch board under your heels to help keep your balance. With your back straight and your head erect, slowly bend your knees until your thighs are parallel to the floor. Go down slowly and back up quickly. As you return to the standing position, try to use only the muscles in your thighs-not your back. And be sure a spotter stands behind you to help with any difficulty you might encounter.

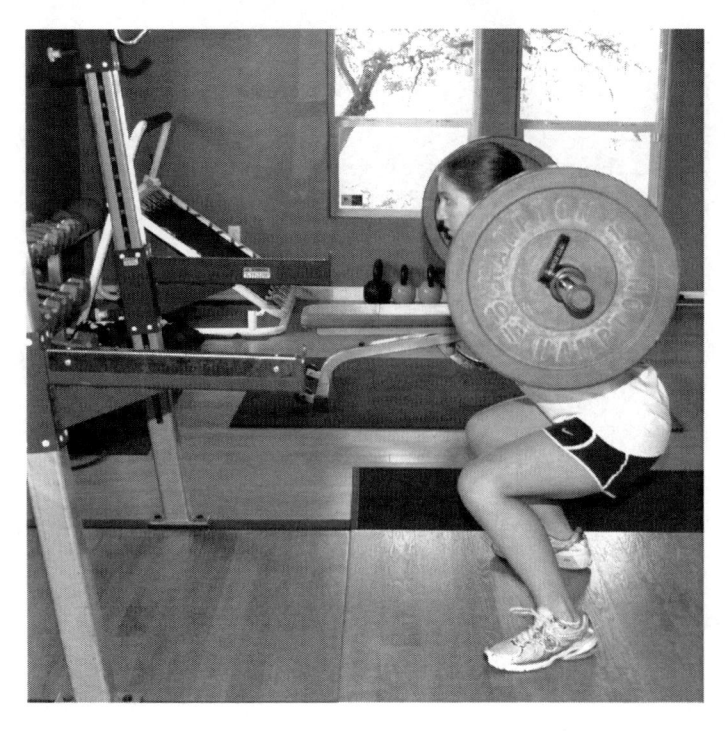

Squat

Bench Presses

Most weight trainers, male and female alike, are partial to this exercise because it strengthens the muscles of the chest and firms the bust-line. Lie on a bench on your back with your feet flat on the floor. Hold the barbell over your chest with your arms straight. Lower the bar until it touches your chest, then press the weight back to starting position.

The bench press has many variations. Some bodybuilders prefer doing the press with dumbbells rather than a barbell because it better isolates the shoulder and chest muscles. Incline presses, which are done on a slanted bench, can be performed using dumbbells or a barbell.

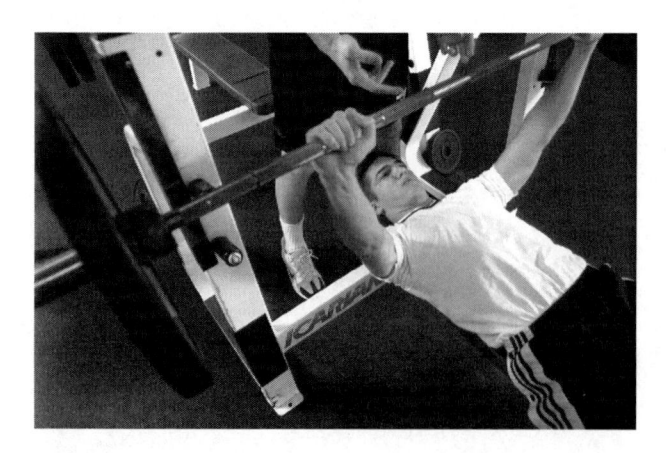

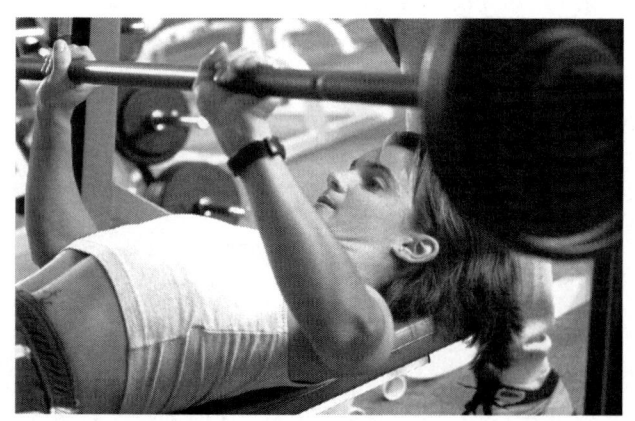

The Bench Press

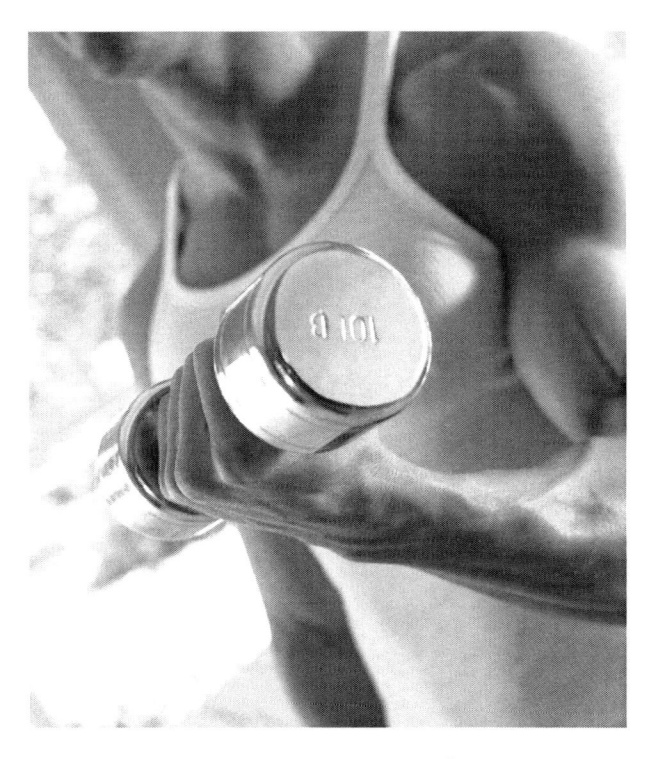

Standing Bicep Curl

Bicep Curls

Grasp a bar with palms up and arms extended. Bend your elbows until the bar reaches your chest. You can perform this exercise with a barbell, dumbbells, or special curl bars, which have bends in the shaft to lessen the strain on the forearms.

Wrist Curls

In a sitting position, rest your forearms on your thighs so that your wrists are lying over your kneecaps, palms up. Grasp the barbell with both hands and let them bend backward. Then bend your wrists upward and slowly return to the starting position. After you get the feel of wrist curls, try the exercise with your palms facing downward.

Pullovers

Lie on a bench or ball with your feet flat on the floor. Rest the barbell on your chest, grasping it with both hands. Slowly lower the bar over your head and behind the edge of the bench, then pull the weight back to your chest. You'll feel the effects of this exercise immediately in your upper and middle back and in your shoulders and arms.

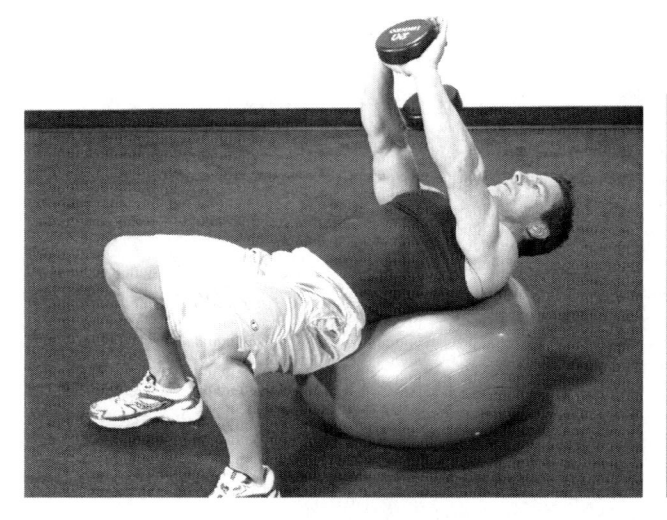

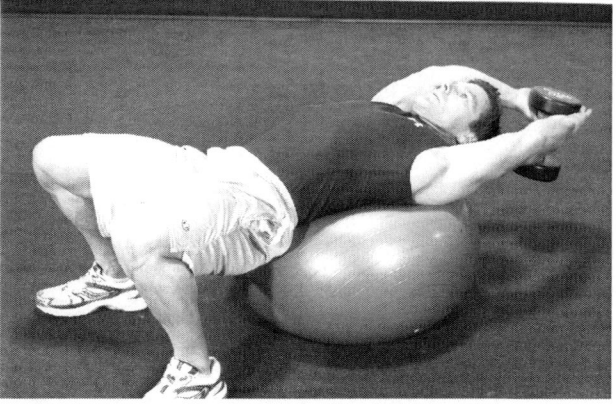

Pullover

THE TRANSITION YEARS

These are only a few of the possible weight training exercises that can be done at home. I suggest you purchase an authoritative guide to weight training, such as my book: (Fahey) *Basic Weight Training for Men and Women*. New York: McGraw Hill, 2003.

Sample Home Strength Program		
Exercise	Repetitions	Sets
1. Sit-Ups	20	1-3
2. Bench Press	10	1-3
3. Squats	10	1-3
4. Shoulder Press	10	1-3
5. Biceps Curls	10	1-3
6. Pullovers	10	1-3
7. Wrist Curls (Palms up and palms down-3 sets each)	10	1-3

The School Physical Education Program

Required physical education is a thing of the past in many areas. This is a very unfortunate situation, especially in view of recent findings that point toward exercise as a vital defense in the battle against heart disease and obesity. We need more exercise in our schools, not less. Today's physical education teachers are well trained and can provide an important service. As a parent, you should fight to keep physical education as part of the core curriculum in the schools.

Americans young and old find themselves with more leisure time every year. Education can provide young people with the ability to use this time in the most enjoyable and beneficial way possible. The schools have the opportunity to introduce sports and recreational activities that young people can carry with them for a lifetime. Adolescence is the time when lifetime habits of exercise and fitness are developed, and the schools should make the most of it.

Often students only have the option of playing team sports such as football and baseball, which require a large number of players. The schools should introduce and stress alternative sports that can become lifetime sports-an adult is much more likely to play tennis, golf, or racquetball than to get twenty people together for a game of football. In addition, the schools should teach the students about how the body works during exercise-muscle chemistry, principles of training, and promote a well-rounded view of sports, exercise, and body chemistry.

Co-ed gym classes are now commonplace in our schools. Adolescents will soon have to deal with the opposite sex in all aspects of daily life; they might as well get used to it with exercise. Integration of the sexes in physical education classes should be flexible enough to allow for ability-grouping to prevent injury, and promote skill development.

Physical education is important for the athlete as well as for the average student. Athletes who plays four years of football or swimming and nothing else may actually graduate from high school recreationally bankrupt, since they never got the chance to develop skills in a variety of lifetime sports. Physical education should give every student exposure to such sports.

Ideally, you should develop a family sports program that complements the physical education program at school. Skills learned at home should reinforce skill learning at school, and vice versa. And remember, physical development cannot be separated from intellectual development. People develop as whole human beings-body and mind are not separate.

Instant Replay

- Adolescence is the period of transition from childhood to adulthood. During this time, children experience an acceleration in growth. Boys tend to improve in physical performance, while girls tend to level off. Gender differences in physical performance are probably due in part to sociological factors.

- Lifetime sports-tennis, racquetball, etc.-should be taught to all adolescents, regardless of whether or not they are athletes. Lifetime habits are acquired during the teen years.

- Endurance is one of the most important parts of fitness because of its contribution to health. The best endurance exercises are running, cycling, swimming, and cross-country skiing. Endurance exercise should be practiced three to five times a week for a minimum of twenty minutes at intensity that increases heart rate from 70 to 85 percent of maximum.

- Heart rate can be used as a built-in speedometer. The training effect occurs at or above the target heart rate. The heart rate during the first ten seconds of recovery after exercise is a good measure of the heart rate during the exercise. Take the pulse for ten seconds and multiply by six.

- Speed and agility can be developed by practicing such exercises as interval training and jumping rope.

- Flexibility or stretching exercises are important for preventing injury and for efficient physical performance. Flexibility exercises should be practiced at least five days a week.

- Strength is important for sports and can be effectively developed during adolescence. Children can improve strength by using their body weight as resistance, or by using weights. For maximum strength development, the child should join a health club or public gymnasium. These facilities usually are better equipped and safer than the home gym.

- Support your high school physical education program. Teenagers need more exercise, not less. An out-of-shape adolescent becomes a hopelessly out-of-shape adult. We are in the midst of a national obesity epidemic that has affected children and adults.

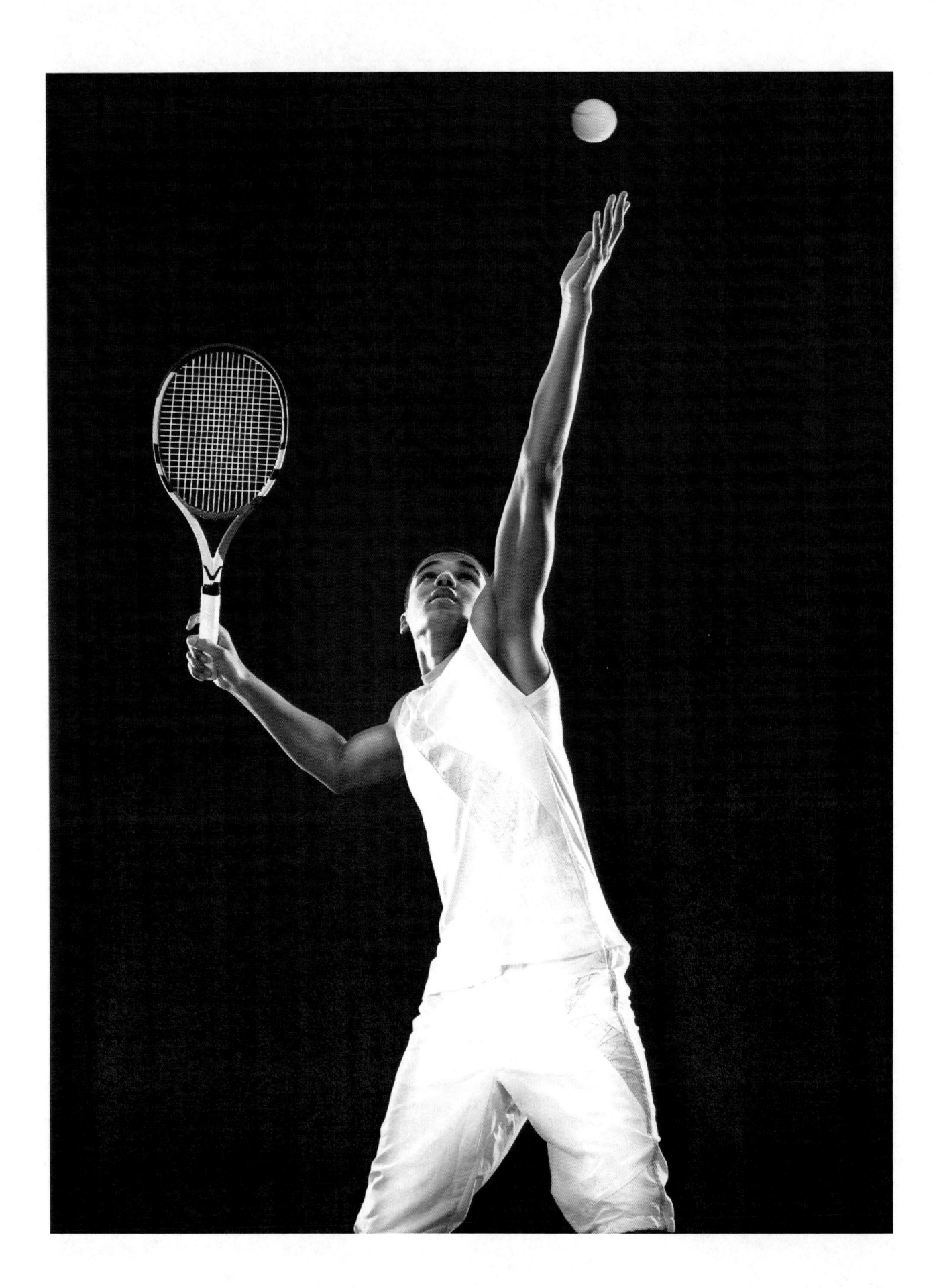

Competitive ATHLETICS

When I first met Keith, he was a freshman in high school. His coordination was extremely poor, but he desperately wanted to be an athlete. His chances looked pretty slim. However, Keith had two things going for him. First, his father was the head football coach of the local college team, and provided Keith with a fitness-oriented environment. Second, he had a burning desire to succeed. He made up his mind that he would train as hard as necessary to get what he wanted.

Keith chose two sports, football and track. His father told him that if he was ever going to make it, he would have to become a lot stronger and a lot quicker. Keith practically moved into the weight room. His early progress was not promising. He had trouble handling his own body weight, let alone barbells. His chest became bruised from doing bench presses. On the playing field, he didn't fare much better than he had the first year. The seniors used Keith as a tackling dummy and seemed to relish stomping over someone so helpless. During track season, he threw the discus 75 feet, a mark that showed very little promise.

Keith kept at it. Throughout the summer he trained harder than ever. Every morning he ran three miles to develop his endurance. Then he played basketball or handball for another couple of hours to increase his speed. He finished in the evening with two hours of heavy weight lifting. When he wasn't practicing his regular workout, he was skipping rope or running windsprints.

Keith continued this vigorous training consistently throughout high school. By the time he was a senior, he had come a long way from the gangling, uncoordinated kid I'd known three years earlier. He had become a tremendous athlete. His arms resembled those on the "Arm and Hammer" baking soda box. He made All-California in football, and placed in the finals of the state track meet in the discus with a throw that exceeded 175 feet. To top his athletic achievements, he got straight A's in his academic subjects throughout his four years of high school. Keith went on to play football at Stanford University and later on a pro-football team. He is now successfully coaching professional football. What did Keith do to gain all of this success? He worked harder than any athlete I've ever seen, and forced himself to be disciplined by making a plan and following it. I am convinced that anyone can become a good athlete if he works hard enough. The trick is to select the right sports, follow the correct training program, and keep

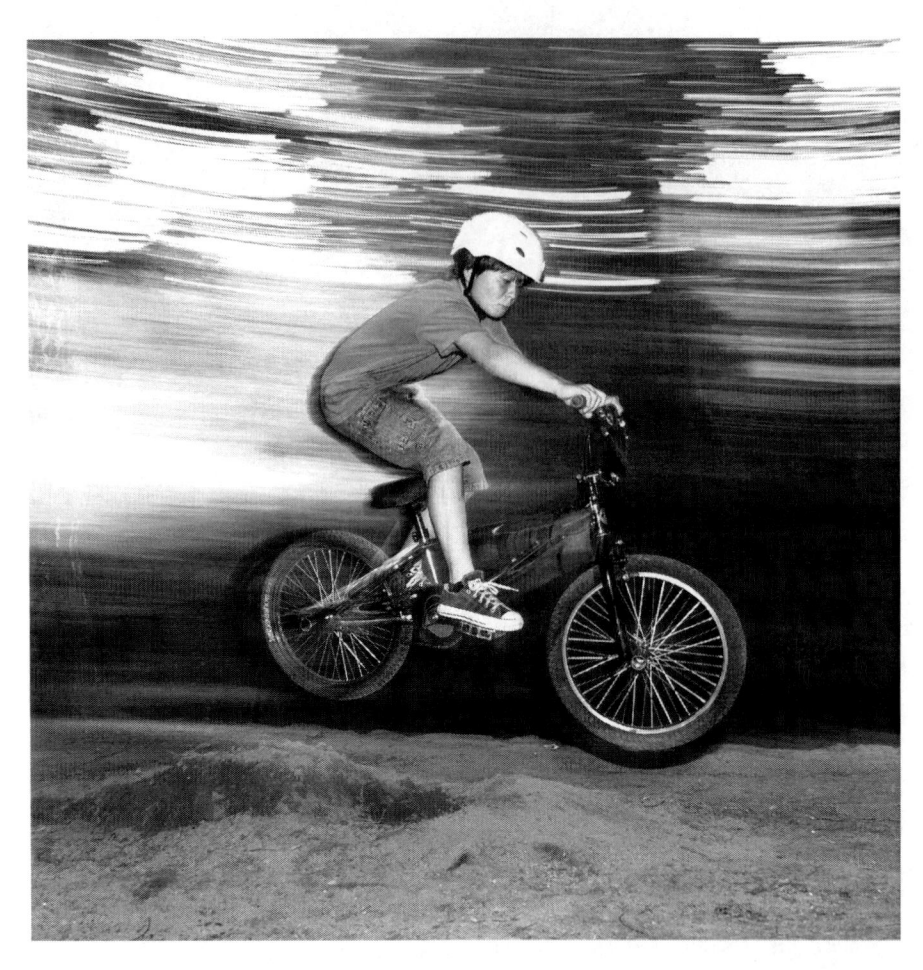

Participation in the right sports will produce an enjoyable athletic experience, along with physical and psychological benefits.

athletic participation psychologically healthy. Athletics can be among the most valuable and cherished experiences in life, whether you become an Olympic gold-medalist or play third string on the high school football team. Parents can help to make athletics a positive experience by providing help and understanding to the young athlete. The essence of parental guidance is the same for both serious and casual participation in sports: helping children achieve their goals in an emotionally healthy environment. To the national-class athlete, this may mean coping with the stress of intense training and competition. To the playground athlete, it may mean developing skills in an atmosphere of fun.

How to Select the Right Sport

It's crucial that children select sports they enjoy. High-level achievement won't be a necessity if the athletic experience is enjoyable,. Participation itself will produce physical and psychological benefits.

Of course, a certain measure of success is usually required for fullest enjoyment in sport. Athletics usually involve the physically gifted, and social pressures exerted on the less skilled and uncoordinated child can be overwhelming. The parents and child should consider the available options and the physical and emotional realities.

Determine the sport in which the child has potential. The gym class is a good proving ground. Can the child run fast? Is he or she bigger or stronger than the other kids? Is he an early or late maturer? Is he good at any one sport in particular? If the child has pretty good sports skills like catching, throwing, and running, he or she may want to consider softball, baseball, basketball, soccer, field hockey (girls), or football (boys). However, if the child does not seem as coordinated as the other kids, then perhaps an alternative such as weight lifting or endurance sports might be more appropriate.

Sports can be divided into three general types: complex movement-oriented sports (basketball, soccer, tennis, and football); fitness-oriented sports (distance running, weight lifting, body building); and technique-oriented sports (discus throwing, gymnastics, diving, golf, etc.). Of course, there is some overlap, but the general categories can help you and the child select the right sports.

Complex movement sports are generally the most popular and most highly regarded in schools, and thus the most competitive. A less skilled child might be better off choosing a sport from one of the other categories. However, this depends on the desires of the child. If a boy has always wanted to be a football player, or a girl a basketball player, don't discourage them. Often, there are junior varsity teams that allow for participation of younger or less skilled children. With training and skill development, the child may do far better than expected.

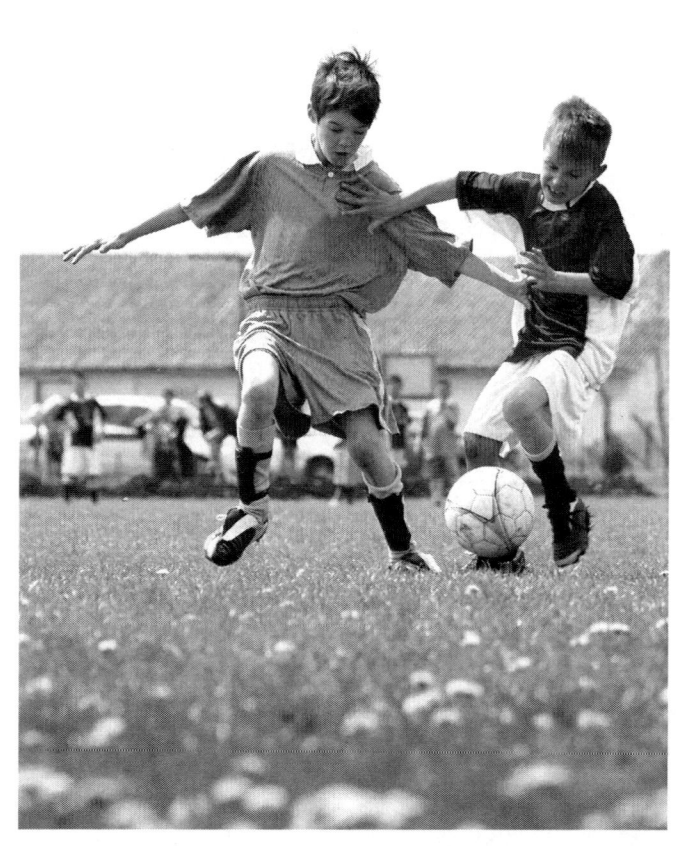

Soccer: a complex movement-oriented sport.

COMPETITIVE ATHLETICS

Fitness-oriented sports offer the less skilled child a chance for some degree of athletic success. Although high levels of success at the national and international levels have certain genetic prerequisites, any child can become extremely proficient in these sports by working hard. Most young athletes don't know the meaning of the term hard work, and thus barely scratch the surface of their potential. Children can't rely on high school track practice or the weight training gym class to make great improvements; they must practice during the summer, during vacations, and on weekends. The key to success in the less skilled youngster is to work harder than the other kids. This requires self-discipline on the part of the child and continued support from parents.

Technique sports offer unique opportunities for athletic success. High achievement on the competitive level in complex technique sports—hammer throwing, equestrian games, diving, gymnastics, and fly casting—requires years of practice, but many of these activities can provide the smaller or less skilled girl or boy with a chance for athletic success that might not be possible in sports like football, basketball, track, or baseball. It's sometimes better to be a big fish in a small pond than to be overwhelmed by the sharks and whales. Willie Sutton, the famous holdup man, was once asked why he robbed banks. He answered, "Because that's where the money is." Technique sports can be where the success is. Participation is the real essence of sport, that participation is much more satisfying if the child is successful and good at the sport.

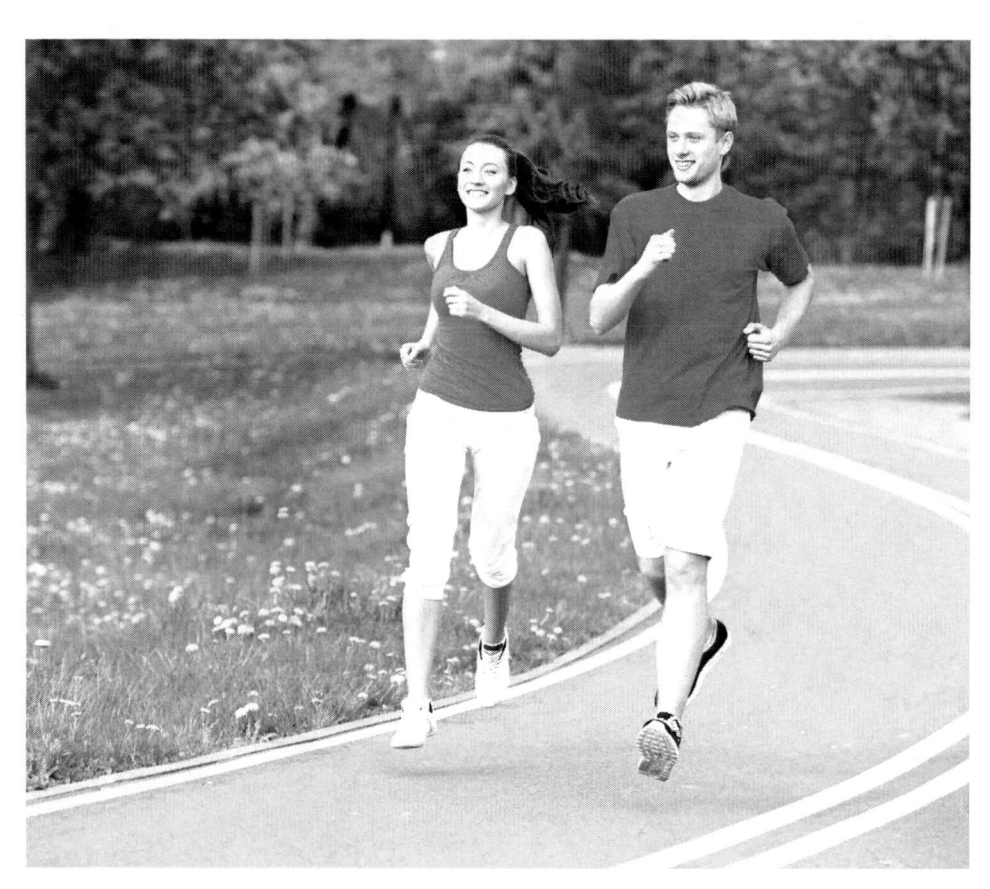

Jogging: a fitness-oriented sport.

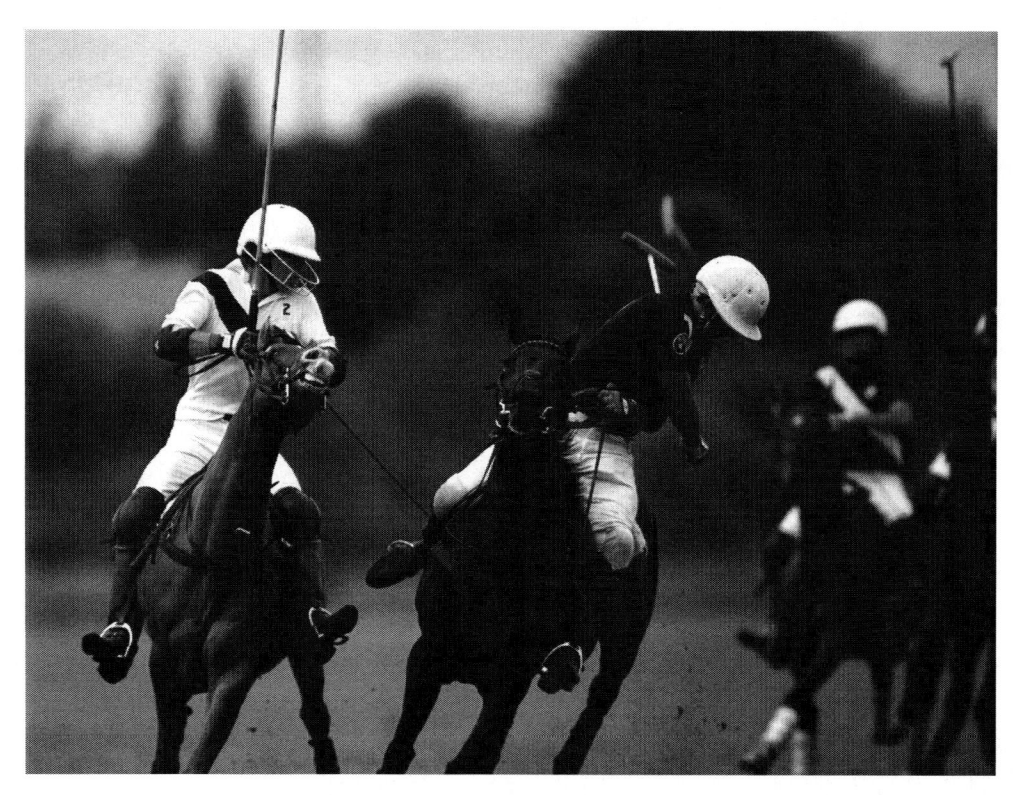

Equestrian sports: technique oriented.

Professional performance analysis can help children assess their potential for various sports and identify their deficiencies he might have. Exercise physiology laboratories can be found in most areas of the country. These facilities exist mainly in large universities, but are now being established as private clinics as well. A word of caution: Don't regard the findings of these labs in absolute terms. Science can help determine sports tendencies, but cannot predict absolute success or failure. Sports medicine can distinguish a child with potential for endurance or speed sports, but does little to predict ability in technique sports.

Years ago, I tested an all-star professional basketball player as part of a publicity campaign. The local newspaper was planning to print a story that compared the pro-basketball player with the average weekend jock. This was the question: How is this all-star professional different from the average guy? We tested both men using common physiological measurements: work capacity and oxygen uptake on the treadmill, body fat and muscle mass, muscle strength and power, flexibility, and muscle fiber type. Each of these tests measures capacity rather than skill.

The findings were startling: The weekend jock performed at almost the same level on most of the tests as the pro player, even though the basketball star was one of the top athletes of his kind in the world. The truth is that the specific skill and fitness of the professional athlete was highly developed for basketball, but lab tests cannot measure specific skills. Laboratory tests can be important for determining athletic capacity, but should not be the only consideration in selecting a sport or trying to predict success.

How Young Should a Child Begin Competition?

The age at which children should begin to compete depends on the nature of their sport. Some sports require specialization at a young age. For example, girls as young as eleven or twelve are Olympic competitors in gymnastics. These girls begin their training at four to six years of age, since early participation may be essential for high-level performance in this sport. Older teenage girls tend to have more fat and wider hips, factors that can be a disadvantage in gymnastics. Recently on television, I saw an extremely skilled ice skater who was only four years old. Other sports, such as football or field events (discus, shotput, hammer and javelin throwing), require a physical maturity for success.

Three questions should be asked by the parents and coaches of prospective young athletes:

1. Is early participation in sports in the interest of the child's emotional and physical health?

2. Will early participation provide the child with an advantage in skill development over other children?

3. Will early athletic participation compromise the child's development in other areas (other sports, social development, music and art appreciation, intellectual development)?

Competition at too early an age can compromise emotional health. Children's sports are sometimes conducted for the benefit and gratification of adults. I'll never forget an experience I had when I was a playground director in San Francisco. An eight-year-old boy was playing second base during a close game. It was a critical part of the baseball sea-

The age which a child should begin to compete depends on the nature of his or her sport.

92 | FITNESS FOR KIDS AND TEENS

son and the boy's team was tied for the lead. A routine pop fly was hit in his direction, and the boy dropped the ball. That was problem enough, but then he made a bad throw to first base, allowing several runs to score. The manager of the team, the father of one of the other boys, became livid with rage:

"You jackass!" he yelled (along with several other expletives). "You just lost the game. The whole season was for nothin' because of you. Get out of my sight—you stink!"

That poor little boy wished he were dead, simply because he had made a human mistake. Of course, such instances are not the norm in children's athletics, but they're common enough. In the past few years, we've seen a parent masquerading a 15 year old boy for a 12-year old and an ice hockey dad killing a coach. Young children are usually not emotionally prepared for the adult standards they might be exposed to in highly structured competitive athletics.

Competitive athletics are not necessarily bad for children under ten. There are outstanding programs in most sports for young children that stress skill development, maximum participation, and fun. As a parent, you should scrutinize the prospective team or athletic club and assess the organizational structure in view of the following:

• Nature of practices. Are they conducted with intelligence, knowledge, and humanity?

• Competitive structure. Do coaches place too much emphasis on winning? Do all the kids get to play, or are the games dominated by the better skilled children? Is too much emphasis placed on awards, all-star games, and championship participation?

• Who are the coaches? Are they professionals who are well trained in skills, teaching, and child development? Or are they parents who seem to be most interested in getting their own kids into the game?

Where skill is concerned, it's doubtful that participation in competitive athletics before the age of eight or ten will give your child the jump on other kids. For boys especially, children need the pubescent growth spurt is develop physical capacity and skill rapidly. Five-to ten-year-olds should only belong to organized teams if those teams provide an atmosphere for learning a variety of movement fundamentals and developing a love of the sport.

Some sports are clearly better than others for young children. For example, gymnastics and soccer provide many opportunities to develop fitness and movement skills, while sports such as tennis and baseball require skills that five- to eight-year-olds don't have. Of course you want your child to learn complex ball-handling skills. But these are developed by practicing specific basic skills, and not necessarily by mere participation in competitive athletics. To become skilled, a child must specialize at some point, but the specialization need not take place before puberty for most sports.

Puberty is the ideal time for specialization. People who begin sports like skiing, tennis, or golf at twenty or twenty-five are at a disadvantage compared to those who begin at twelve. Usually the gap cannot be breached, regardless of how much the older person practices. Sports scientists have long been interested in determining the stages of development in which the potential for improving in skill and capacity is greatest.

Are Athletics Physically Safe?

Organized sports for children, particularly junior level football and baseball, have received a lot of bad press in recent years, but much of this criticism is unjustified. High school and college football have been extensively criticized because of the risk of serious injuries, and many people extrapolate these dangers youth football. The argument goes like this: If football is a dangerous sport for high school and college players, then it must be even worse for young children with growing bones. Statistically, the injury rate in young football players is much lower than in high school or college players. Young children are smaller, slower, and generally less aggressive than older players. Junior level players can't generate the power or generate tremendous the forces that cause serious injuries in the older players.

Children's sports are safe if precautions are taken. In Chapter 5, I will discuss ways of preventing athletic injuries.

Getting the Child Involved in Competitive Athletics

There are well-defined pathways for entry, participation, and eventual success in most sports. Usually, a child begins sports participation in school, by joining a club, or by taking lessons. Schools stress football, basketball, baseball, and track and field, so this is a logical starting place for playing these sports. There are also junior levels for these sports, though it is doubtful that competitive experience gained before age twelve is required or even desirable for later success. Before this age, emphasize fitness and helping the children improve basic movement skills, such as throwing, catching, running, agility, and balance.

The best way to learn about opportunities for competitive school sports for children younger than twelve is to ask the coaches of the local junior high or high school. They will know where to find programs that provide good experiences. You can also contact your local recreation department, police athletic league, or YMCA for information.

Sports such as swimming, gymnastics, equestrian games, canoeing, bobsledding, downhill skiing, and karate are not popular school sports, so children must join a club or take lessons and may involve considerable expense. Track for children under twelve can be considered a club sport, too. Success in these sports requires the competition, training, and coaching that only a club can provide.

How to Choose the Right Sports Club

Select sports clubs according to these criteria:

• Aspiration and skill of the child. Some clubs are geared to the national-class athlete and are much too intimidating for the average child. A beginning miler will be blown away if he tries to run the fifteen or twenty 440-yard dashes

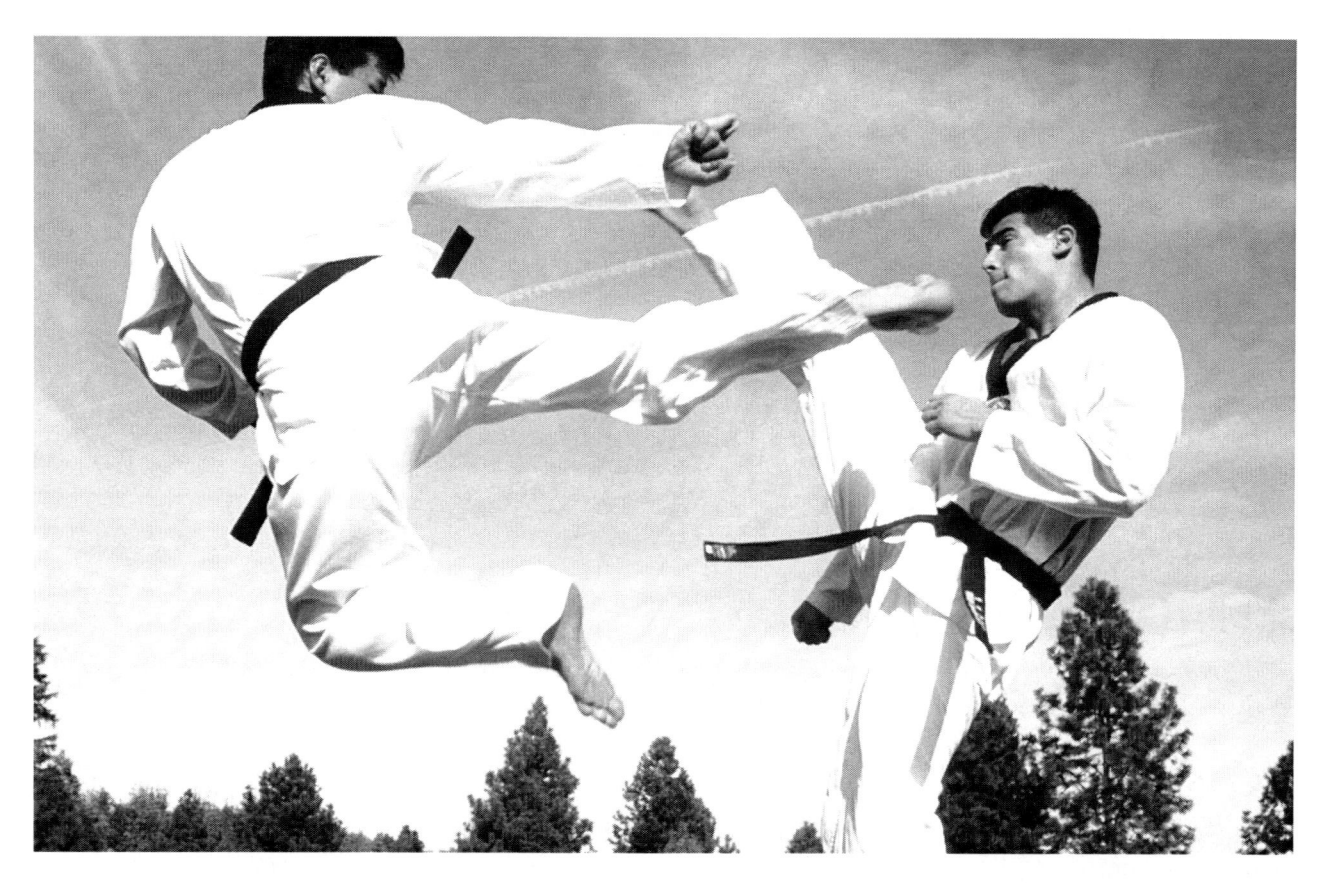

Karate: becoming proficient usually requires professional lessons and considerable expense.

practiced by the national-class runner in 60 to 80 seconds.

A beginner might first choose a less competitive club. The workouts will generally be less severe, and the level of competition will be lower. If the child shows an interest in more vigorous competition and more challenging workouts, then it's time for a change. Don't pressure children. Try to make athletics a positive experience. High-level performance is very difficult in unchallenging environments, so if a more competitive club serves the needs of the child, move on.

• Family circumstances. Membership in top sports clubs costs a lot of money—directly and indirectly. Usually, there are only one or two swim or track clubs that serve a large geographical area. Engaging in top-level competition may require the child to commute hundreds of miles every week. This costs money and time. I've known several athletes who spend three hours a day on the road getting to and from practice. This kind of time commitment can cause severe family problems. Is the sport that important for the child? How much will participation in a top club disrupt the family? Are you being fair to the non-athletes in the family?

Some sports can be extremely expensive. In skiing, for example, the $1000 to $3000 investment in skis, boots, clothes, helmet, etc., is just a drop in the bucket compared to the travel expenses and coaching fees. Today's young competitive skiers usually board at ski resorts, where they can go to school and train. During the summer, it's a good idea to go to Argentina or New Zealand for training. That's the kind of commitment required for success in that sport. Participation in competitive horseback riding can be just as costly. In addition to purchasing and maintaining your horse, you have to provide the funds for travel and entry fees. Tennis and golf require many years of expensive lessons to develop finely honed skills.

• Club philosophy. Scrutinize the philosophy of the coaching staff. Do the coaches view athletics as a vehicle for child development or as a means of racking up an impressive win-loss record? Are the coaches good examples for your child? Even in today's permissive society, a child shouldn't have as a model a coach who swears, smokes, is abusive to officials, and doesn't treat people with respect.

I don't think that an emphasis on winning is a bad thing, so long as it's kept in its proper perspective. You'll have to look hard and long to find a coach who doesn't want to win. Winning and the will to win are important components of sport—remove these and all you have left is play. However, the coaches' main emphasis should be on excellence rather than on winning or losing. Anyone can "win" if he has the right opponent—someone less developed or less skilled. If children strive for excellence, they will win at higher and higher levels of competition. Winning without emphasis on excellence is meaningless.

Ideally, sports should be played for their intrinsic value. In this context, the winning experience will be one of pride for a job well done. On the other hand, a meaningless win leaves a child asking, "Is that all there is?"

How Should the Parent Deal with the Coach?

Coaches are like anybody else—some are shy, others are aggressive. Most are dedicated, but some are just putting the time in and waiting for retirement. Children have to learn to deal with the different personalities of their coaches. Interpersonal relationships are never easy. When I coached children's teams, there were some kids who didn't like me and other kids with whom I had a great relationship. It's the same with all coaches—they're only human. Some personality clashing with coaches is natural. The parent shouldn't run to the coach every time the child feels a little threatened, underestimated, or unappreciated; the child won't always be able to depend on his parents to solve his problems. He must learn to cope with them himself, provided the coach is not practicing unprofessional behavior. Most coaches are extremely knowledgeable and dedicated, and it's disrespectful and unfair to undermine his authority or criticize him behind his back.

There may be times when the coach's behavior subjects your child to physical or emotional harm. Practices such as withholding water from children, promoting the use of anabolic steroids or amphetamines, physical or emotional abuse, or prodding athletes to play when injured should not be tolerated. In these cases, the coach should be directly confronted. If that doesn't do any good, then take stronger measures.

Let coaches do their job. Although it's important to support your child and offer help when it's needed, let the coach worry about training schedules and competitive strategies. Coaching strategies differ very little in any given sport. The most important factor is the child himself; if he works very hard and has some talent, he will be successful. If your kid doesn't get to play first string in field hockey or football, it may be that he or she is less skilled than the others. Don't automatically blame the coach; instead, encourage your child to work harder. Remember, few coaches will deliberately play a less skilled child in place of a superior player. Rely on the coach's objectivity and sense of fair play.

Maximizing Your Child's Sports Experience

Children will usually specialize in specific sports by the time they're 10-16 years old. Parents can't force children to like sports. But once a child has shown an interest, there are many things you can do to help make the athletic experience positive.

The Emotional Elements

The child is the one involved in the sports program, not you. Don't try to relive your dreams through children. They should be central in the decision-making process regarding their sports participation. Some mistakes are inevitable, but so is some measure of success. So, let the child do it!

Consider the child's motivation. Not everyone wants to be an Olympic champion. Some kids just want to be part of a group or to be with their friends. For these children, participation in athletics is valuable even though they may not achieve great success or skill.

Don't overreact to the situation. If the child expresses a desire to be a ski racer, don't run out the next day to buy $2000 worth of equipment and clothing. Children often don't know what they really want. Provide opportunities for participation; if the child demonstrates sincerity and a real desire to become proficient, then spend the money on equipment. Once child are seriously involved in sports, they should have the best equipment the family can afford. Competitive sports are difficult enough without the athlete being hampered by poor equipment.

Providing emotional support is one of your most important responsibilities. It's very difficult kids to sit on the bench or perform poorly. Let the child know that you understand the problem. Provide guidance—sometimes a child may want to quit the team when things get tough. They should learn to stick it out and overcome adversity. A little understanding and direction can often keep the athletic experience in its proper perspective for children.

The Physical Aspects

Give the child the benefit of your experience and maturity. Usually, children only want to spend time on the aspects of the sport they enjoy. If you encourage an intelligent approach to training and practice, you will help the child develop into a proficient, well-rounded athlete.

Staying in Shape

Encourage the child to stay in shape all year. Most athletic programs, except at the highest levels of competition, do not stress excellence. This is understandable. Most athletic children have other interests besides sports, and probably wouldn't tolerate a high-powered program. However, children should train all year if they are really serious about sports. Most improvements in performance are made during the off-season. For example, a girl can expect to make relatively little progress on the balance beam during an eight-week gymnastics season. However, her improvement could be substantial if she developed her technique over a twelve-month period.

Speed and strength are two factors of physical fitness that can turn a relatively unskilled football player into a "studly bear-cat" within a year. When you're in good shape, you don't get tired—your skill level can remain high for the whole game.

The child who trains only part of the year has to spend many weeks getting into shape once the season begins. Athletes who are already in shape at the start of the season, will be better athletes once competition begins.

Training

Encourage children to develop basic fundamentals. Most kids would rather play games than work on drills. Although games are a great way of developing some skills, they tend to reinforce bad habits. In tennis, if children practice serves, ground strokes, cross-court and line shots, they will have a repertoire of basic skills that will make them very effective in competition. Practice sessions should offer the opportunity to refine skills that may be difficult to develop in a game.

Encourage children to work hard and to approach the sport intelligently. For example, good football coaches have their practice time organized to the minute. They place emphasis on weaknesses and on efficient execution of the most important factors of the game. Likewise, children should concentrate on weaknesses and on the most important skills of the sport.

Emphasize consistency in the training program. Improve fitness by systematically increasing the difficulty of the workout. An athlete may only be capable of bench pressing 65 pounds today, but by consistently increasing the severity of the workout, the lift could be 300 pounds in a couple of years. Strong bodies don't usually happen by accident. They are built through hard work.

Children should keep a training diary. A plain notebook will serve the purpose nicely. The child should record the type of workouts, feelings about performance, short-term and long-term goals, diet, weight, and height. A training diary will help with long-term planning and will add greater structure and purpose to the training program.

Practices should concentrate on the most important aspects of the sport. I knew a young basketball player who practiced in the gym near my laboratory. She worked very hard, but her practices were very inefficient. She spent most of her time working on free throws from the foul line and set shots. Motor learning scientists have found that the learning curves for these skills are almost flat; excessive practice does little to develop further skill. June should have worked on other skills, such as dribbling, jump shots, and lay-ups that would make her more effective as a player.

I observed a junior level football team that also had very inefficient practice sessions. The kids spent the first three weeks of training on calisthenics and pre-game warm-up exercises. They looked like a precision drill team during the warm-ups. The whole team yelled the repetition number in perfect unison and clapped at the same time during the jumping jacks. But they played very poor football. Their execution of plays was extremely sloppy, and reflected their lack of practice. The team didn't work on what was important. They had the best pre-game warm-ups in the league, but the newspaper failed to mention that after their weekly losses.

Keeping Sports in the Proper Perspective

A fifteen-year-old boy or girl may think nothing of playing basketball with damaged knee ligaments. Children at that age usually find it difficult to picture all the pain in store when they turn thirty-five and arthritis sets in. Anabolic steroids may seem to a high school student like a good way to improve strength, but the side effects may be detrimental when the child becomes an adult. Athletes should learn a variety of sports skills that will allow them to continue exercising when they retire from competitive athletics.

Athletes should develop and maintain other interests to make them well-rounded people. Even the most gifted athlete who puts all his eggs in one basket will eventually be in for a rude awakening. Professional and Olympic sports will never be more than a dream for most children. In the United States, where there are over 300 million people, only about ten thousand make their living as professional athletes. Even if a kid does make it to the top, how long is he going to stay there? For every athlete who continue to play well into their forties, there are thousands of hopeful kids who fail to make it at eighteen or twenty. Children need a varied educational experience so that they can be educated members of society. Few athletes will end up playing sports professionally.

Sports Camps

Camps are available for most sports. They range from summer ski racing clinics in South America to day camps at the local recreation center. Many of these camps are excellent; they teach aspiring young athletes fundamental skills that are essential for success. Others are rip-offs, leaving in their wake many disappointed and disillusioned youngsters. I once heard a professional athlete remark, "I made a fortune from a sports camp, and I only showed my face for twenty minutes." Many athletic stars lend their names to sports summer camps knowing that the parents of idolizing children will shell out several hundred dollars in the hope of receiving expert instruction for the child.

Other camps give good value for the money. For example, Olympic throwers John Powell and Brian Old field put on throwing camps at Dennison University in Ohio every summer. They are present every minute of the camp and spend long hours working with youngsters. I am extremely impresses with the quality of coaching and their level of professionalism. There are many valuable camps such as this, so check around.

• Before signing up your son or daughter for one of these camps, do some checking: Are you getting good value for your dollar? Camps can be expensive. Make sure they have the facilities and staff that they advertise. If a star athlete is used as a drawing card, find out if he will participate in coaching or if he's just a figurehead.

• Is the level of competition and skill at the camp appropriate for the child? A camp for champion-caliber tennis players will be inappropriate for a child who has just started the game.

• Does the child really want to go? Don't push children to go to a camp if they don't want to go. Sports should be a positive experience. Also, sports camps can be a lot more fun if they go with a friend.

You can learn about sports camps through college physical education departments, YMCAs, recreation centers, sports clubs, scouts, and magazines. Specialty magazines for sports like skiing, tennis, mountain climbing, and football can often provide additional information. Sunset magazine, for instance, maintains a directory of summer camps.

Science and Athletics

America has the most advanced knowledge of sports medicine in the world. There has been more progress in exercise physiology during the past ten years than in all of history. Old myths have been cast aside. The big problem is getting the information from the lab to the athlete.

The Sports Science Myth

Before the fall of communism in Eastern Europe, the small country of East Germany won as many medals as the great world powers, the United States and Russia. The media reported rumors of "secret labs" in East Germany and mysterious potions that led to athletic victory. The general feeling was that the East German scientists knew something that ours didn't. There is no evidence, though, to support this idea. Although we now know that they gave many of their athletes steroids, the East Germans were simply better organized than we were. Actually, their information and techniques was not as advanced as ours, but they used what they had very well. Because of their political system, they could select athletes who showed promise and developed them systematically by using the principles in this book on a national scale.

Science has contributed tremendously to the improved performances seen in the last twenty years. Athletes have become faster, stronger, more skilled, and attain more endurance at a faster rate than at any time in history. These achievements have not only affected equipment and playing surfaces, but training methods as well. Athletes and coaches should be aware of the latest information in order to make practice sessions as effective as possible.

Equipment and Playing Surfaces

Space-age plastics and synthetics have revolutionized equipment in many sports. In pole vaulting, for instance, new materials have enabled competitors to vault more than twenty feet. It was only 50 years ago that Dutch Warmerdam was practically immortalized for vaults slightly over fifteen feet. People haven't changed that much, but the modern fiberglass pole is a lot different than Warmerdam's bamboo pole. Technological advances have redefined other sports as well. New running track surfaces make all-weather training possible and maximize traction for faster times. Tennis racquets are lighter and made of materials that allow more control of the ball. Ski manufacturers produce equipment that is designed for specific terrains and ability levels—a long way from the hickory boards and bear claw bindings of 50 years ago. Discuses are designed with weight on the outside so they'll spin faster and go farther if thrown correctly. Heart rate monitors allow runners to more accurately assess training levels and maximize efficiency. Running shoes are designed with a consideration for the mechanics and anatomy of the foot. In today's world of sports, a young athlete is at a disadvantage without up-to-date equipment.

Advances in Training

Training has evolved from a hit-or-miss proposition into a science. Sports scientists continue to isolate specific factors of fitness, and to design and update training regimens. Beginning in the 1950s, weight training was incorporated into the training programs for football, track and field, and wrestling. This has resulted in rapid strength gains that have had a tremendous effect on the caliber of play. Today, specialized weight training programs improve performance in women's and men's swimming, baseball, softball, volleyball, skiing, and water polo.

Exercise machines have also been advanced dramatically. Contemporary devices develop strength through the use of the full range of motion of various body areas. These machines also strengthen muscle groups that are difficult to develop with barbells. The exercise machines of the past were difficult to use and were not as effective for isolating muscle groups.

Biomechanics, the study of efficient movement techniques, has evolved from an art form to a science. The application of biomechanics in sports has great potential for improving movement. Techniques, such as the rotary shot-put style and the "Fosbury flop" high jump, have resulted in substantial improvements in performance. Computer analysis of sports performance will soon be available to the average athlete, and will facilitate a faster rate of improvement and more efficient techniques. Computers and video cameras are essential coaching tools.

Ergogenic Aids

Ergogenic aids are substances that improve performance. Throughout history, athletes and warriors have sought out substances that would improve strength, speed, and endurance. The ancients often ate the liver of a fallen enemy whose bravery they admired, in the hope of becoming braver themselves. Modern athletes have experimented with such substances as anabolic steroids, growth hormone, blood supplements, creatine monohydrate, amphetamines, vitamins, bee pollen, oxygen, and protein supplements. Most so-called ergogenic aids either don't work or are unhealthy.

Anabolic steroids are chemical drugs produced through laboratory synthesis. Many athletes use steroids to increase body weight, strength, and endurance, since the chemicals act to duplicate the muscle-building properties of the male hormone testosterone. In fact, a large number of successful athletes in such strength-oriented sports as discus, shot-put, and weight lifting use steroids to enhance physical gains. The use of these drugs is unwise for older athletes, but in teenagers it can be disastrous. Anabolic steroids have been found to cause the long bones of the arms and legs to fuse prematurely, thus curtailing further growth. In addition, the chemicals may be toxic to the liver and may be related to the development of prostate or liver cancer. They can also cause acne, abnormal hair growth, and a deceleration of sperm production. In girls, steroids can produce masculinization and affect the ability to have children. The best advice you can give to a teenager is not to take these drugs—the benefits are questionable and there are definite health risks.

Anabolic steroids do improve strength and increase muscle mass — if you take enough of them.

Protein supplements are very popular with those teenage boys who want desperately to increase their muscle mass. They reason that if muscles are made of proteins, then increasing the protein content of the diet will increase muscle size. Unfortunately, it doesn't work that way. The body only needs about 1-1.5 grams of protein per kilogram of body weight; any additional protein is used to fuel metabolism. New studies show that taking protein supplements immediately before weight training may speed muscle growth. However, it's not known if this practice is effective over the long run. The best way to increase muscle bulk is to work very hard in the weight room. Money spent on protein supplements is better spent on sports equipment.

Vitamin supplements rival or surpass protein in popularity as an ergogenic aid. Vitamin C has been credited with everything from curing the common cold to improving endurance. In moderate doses, the vitamin is not dangerous. Vitamin E is believed by some to increase endurance. It became popular when it was discovered to increase sexual potency in roosters. Human roosters latched onto the possibilities and made some lucky vitamin manufacturers rich. The vast majority of scientific research studies, though, have failed to find a link between Vitamin E and improved endurance. In fact, recent clinical evidence suggests that high doses (above 1000 international units) may cause lethargy and loss of energy in some people. Vitamin B12 is popular with weight lifters who believe it increases muscle size. Any benefit is probably the result of a placebo effect—the athlete believes it works and so it does, even though the drug has no reliable physiological effect. Usually the only harm these vitamins do is to the pocketbook. However, fat-soluble Vitamins A and D can be toxic because they are stored in fat and build up to high levels in the body.

Blood boosting via a drug called EPO is another ergogenic aid. EPO promotes large increases in work capacity and maximal oxygen consumption. Blood doping increases the oxygen-carrying capacity of blood and improves endurance. The drug is linked to many deaths in endurance athletes in Europe. Amphetamines and cocaine are dangerous drugs that are often abused in athletics. Although they may increase performance in some endurance sports, they mask fatigue and hamper performance in sports requiring judgment. These drugs can interfere with the physiology of the heart, and have caused deaths in endurance events like the Tour de France bicycle race. Their use has no place in sports.

The use of oxygen to speed up recovery was popularized by the Japanese swimming team in the 1936 Olympics. Many people attributed their success to their use of oxygen between races. Numerous scientific studies have shown that breathing pure oxygen has no real effect on recovery. However, the use of oxygen during recovery remains popular simply because it's practiced by several professional football teams. If you could breathe pure oxygen during exercise, it might help, but that's not allowed in any sport I know of except scuba diving or assaults on Mt. Everest.

Creatine monohydrate supplements are very popular with young athletes because they increase strength, muscle mass, and help speed recovery from intense exercise. Most studies show that the supplement is effective and safe. However, some athletes and coaches report problems with muscle cramping. We don't know the long-term effects in children, so this supplement is not recommended.

The very idea of using ergogenic aids is contrary to the values sports should promote in young people. Furthermore, most ergogenic aids are illegal in competitive sports. Sports should teach children to work hard and succeed on the basis of their own accomplishments. Young athletes shouldn't think that all you need to do to win is take a pill.

Nutrition and Athletics

Good nutritional habits should be established during childhood. Children should be encouraged to eat meals that are low in saturated fats. Stay away from fried foods, meat fat, and junk food. Protein intake is important but shouldn't be overemphasized. Carbohydrates are just as important to good athletic performance.

Carbohydrates, which are stored in muscles and the liver as glycogen, are the most important fuel for high intensity muscular work. Low glycogen stores decrease performance. The symptoms commonly associated with overtraining—poor performance, chronic fatigue, a dead feeling in your muscles—can sometimes be directly related to a low level of glycogen. Endurance athletes, particularly, should be on a high-performance diet that contains 60 to 70 percent carbohydrates. Foods like grains, cereals, fruits, bread, potatoes, beans, and corn are better sources of carbohydrates than foods high in simple sugar.

Girls and Athletics

Women and girls have many opportunities in sports today. Athletics are a critical part of the education of all children. As a parent, you should insist that your daughter (or, for that matter, anyone's daughter) gets an equal opportunity for athletic participation.

Girls should receive the same quality of coaching as boys, but forcing boys and girls to play on the same team is probably not a good idea. Teenage boys are usually physically superior to teenage girls. If there is only one team and it's coed, most girls won't get a chance to play. If a girl is good enough to play on a boys' team, she should have the opportunity to do so; otherwise, there should be a girls' team for her to play on. Girls' teams, however, should not be forced to play on second-rate fields or discriminated against in any other way.

A Price to Pay

Athletics can be the most positive and enjoyable experience of a lifetime. The young athlete develops friendships and cultivates psychological benefits that will stay with him or her for many years to come. An unavoidable part of athletics, however, is competition, and competition can crush a child who can't cope with it. I've seen athletes, both young and old, give up almost everything to win, only to have their hopes shattered. The agony of defeat can break a person, but you must teach your child to shake it off and move on to something else, or try again.

There is a price to pay for both success and failure in athletics, but with the proper mental attitude a child can cope with both. The parent can help keep things in their proper perspective by encouraging a healthy attitude:

• Teach the child that winning or losing has little to do with his being a person. If he loses, he's not a bum, and if he wins, he's not better than everybody else.

• Children must sacrifice if they want to be successful. Top performance in any sport requires long hours of training. Everybody who makes it to the Olympics has worked hard. The secret of success in athletics is to work hard, train intelligently, get a good coach, and make the most of natural ability and luck.

• Always do your best. As Bear Bryant, the great football coach, said, "My 90-percent player playing 100 percent will beat your 100-percent ball player playing 90 percent every time." Concentrate on what you're doing. Leave nothing to chance; if you have a weakness, correct it.

• Be in the best possible condition. An out-of-shape athletes are in trouble, no matter how skilled they are. There is a price to pay for being in top shape. The dividends appear in the win column.

• Learn from your mistakes. Analyze your technique and try to become as efficient as possible. The more wasted motion you can eliminate, the better you'll perform.

Bill of Rights for Young Athletes*

The National Association of Sports and Physical Education has outlined the basic rights of boys and girls involved in athletics:

- Right of the opportunity for participation in sports -regardless of ability level
- Right to participate at a level that is commensurate with each child's development level
- Right to have qualified adult leadership
- Right to participate in safe and healthy environments
- Right of each child to share in the leadership and decision-making of their sports participation
- Right to play as a child and not as an adult
- Right to proper preparation for participation in the sport
- Right to an equal opportunity to strive for success
- Right to be treated with dignity by all involved
- Right to have fun through sport

Reprinted with permission from the National Association of Sports and Physical Education.

Instant Replay

- Hard work and dedication are the great equalizers in athletics. The child who consistently puts forth a good effort will eventually realize success.

- Success and enjoyment in athletics require selecting the right sport. Selection should be based on preference, talent, body size, family finances, and the availability and practicality of the sport.

- Early competition is usually not in the best interest of children. Sports participation before age twelve should stress the development of basic movement skills and fundamentals, rather than competition.

- Parents should encourage the child to develop the best possible physical condition and maintain it all year long.

- Parents should help children keep athletics in their proper perspective. Shortsighted decisions may be regretted later in life. Encourage your child to develop intellectually and socially as well as athletically.

- Sports medicine and science can help your child improve. Modern developments in equipment and training methods will enhance performance and enjoyment in the future.

- Girls should have the same opportunities for athletic participation as boys.

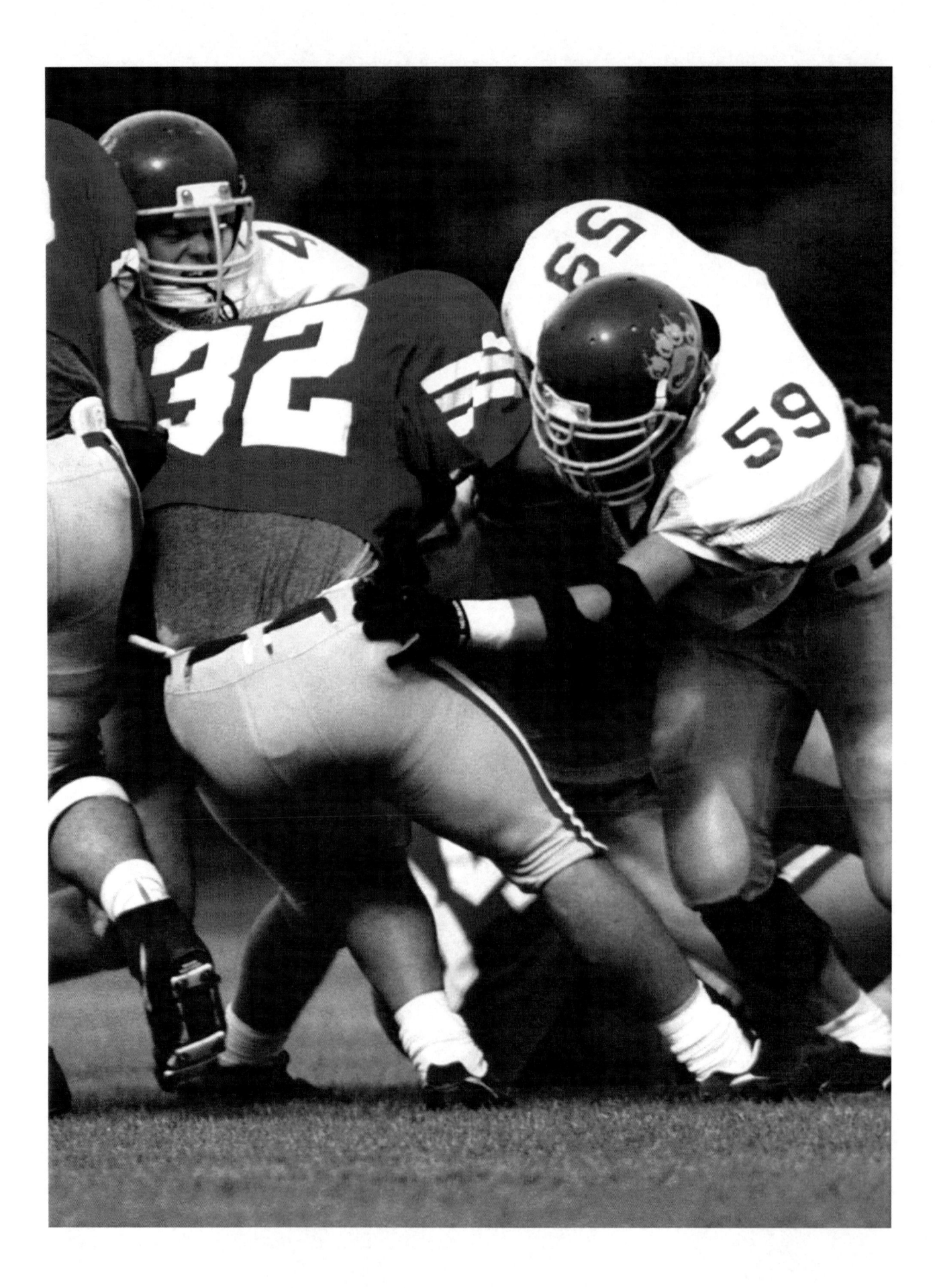

Athletic INJURIES

PREVENTION AND TREATMENT

It was first down and ten yards to go on the Oakdale Vikings' own 30-yard line. Jim Haynes was the quarterback, and he was having a great year. Only two more games and the season would be over—Jim was sure to get tons of scholarship offers from the big schools. He took the snap, dropped back into a pocket of blockers, and looked for an open receiver. But things started to go wrong—Jim's pass protection deteriorated, and he was forced into the open with several defensive players breathing down his neck. All of a sudden a blitzing linebacker came at him like the night train. Jim went down hard as the linebacker hit him with a crunch on the side of his knee. The knee seemed to snap like a rubber band. Jim's season—and possibly his career—was over.

Scenes like this are repeated time and again on playing fields across the country. There are risks involved in athletics, but most of us feel the risks are worth it, in light of the many benefits of sports. However, coaches, athletes, and parents should all take steps to minimize athletic injuries and to make sure they're adequately rehabilitated when they do occur.

Athletics can be one of the profound influences in a child's life. But if an athletic program presents undue risk of serious injury, it may produce an adult with chronically sore joints and lack of function. A safe athletic program requires physicians, coaches, athletes, trainers, and parents to work together in an organized manner to insure that sports participation is a positive experience, and not one that produces athletic casualties. This chapter summarizes the prevention and treatment of athletic injuries in children's sports.

Preventing Injuries

Promoting physical fitness is the best way to prevent injury in children's sports. Other factors critical for injury prevention include proper coaching, good equipment, and adequate medical supervision.

Proper Coaching

Coaches are in a unique position because they can shape the physical and, to an extent, the emotional condition of their team members.

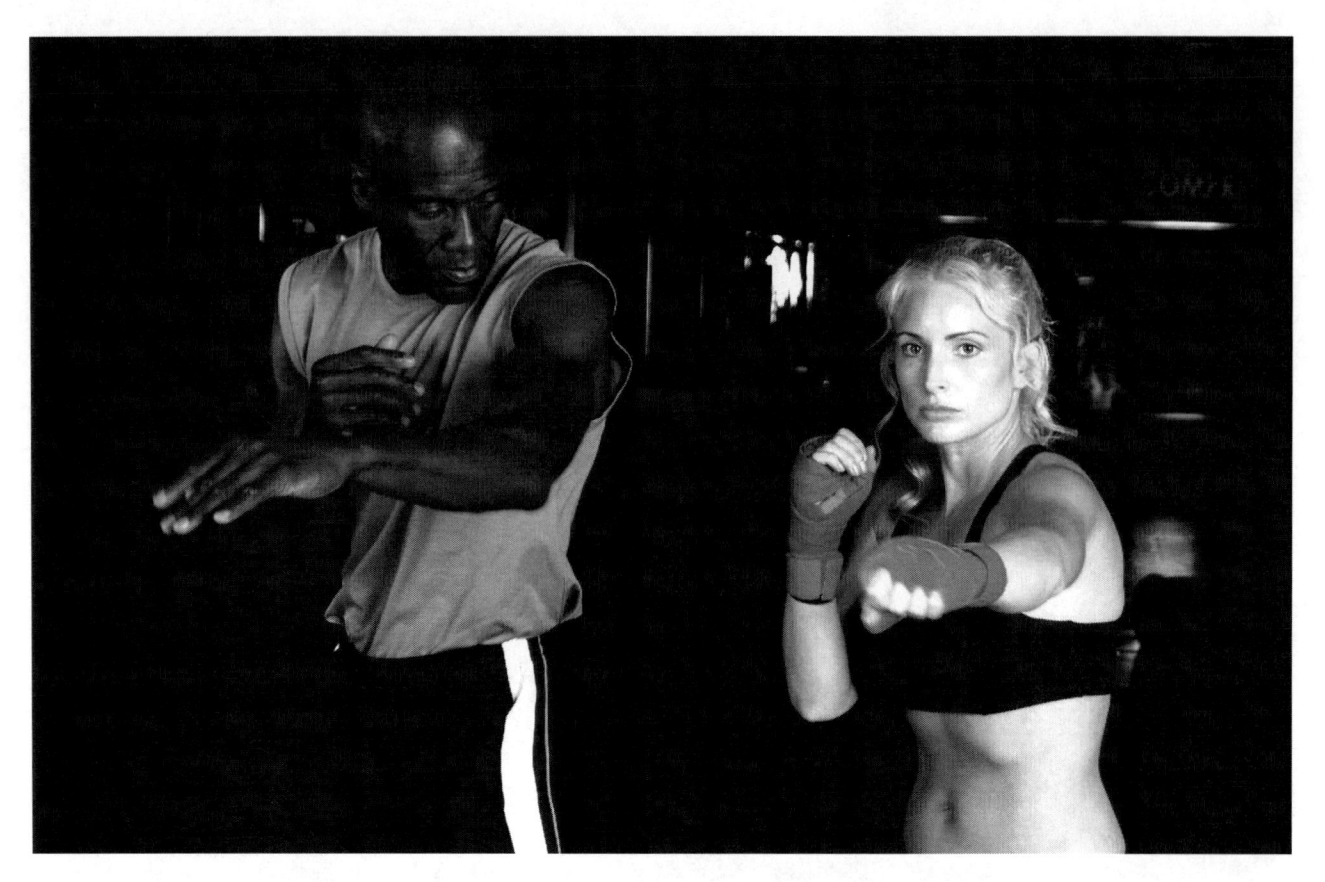

Let the coach do his job. He can minimize the possibility of injury by teaching proper fundamentals.

Coaches sets the tone of the practices and games. They decide whether they'll be vicious or sportsmanlike, sloppy or played with finesse.

Most coaches are knowledgeable and extremely dedicated. They teach techniques that prevent injuries and they encourage a high degree of physical conditioning. And they keep up to date with current knowledge of training and exercise physiology.

A good coach can minimize even minor injuries by teaching proper sports fundamentals. For example, coaches can reduce the risk of shoulder and elbow injuries by teaching proper throwing techniques.. They can reduce back injuries by showing athletes sound lifting methods. Good sports fundamentals make movements more efficient and predictable—it's the unexpected that often results in injury. Most children will participate in sports in "sandlots" if they don't have the opportunity to participate in organized athletics. Sandlot games are notorious for causing serious injuries. I remember several instances from my own childhood—one boy was in a body cast for six months after a playground tackle football game, and another broke his neck and became a quadriplegic from an impromptu game of rugby. Good coaches can minimjze tragic injuries by teaching children proper fundamentals and practice according to the rules.

The coaches' attitude are important in preventing injuries. Coaches deal with impressionable boys and girls. Coaches who tell young players to "kill" the opponent or uses unsportsmanlike behavior can expect their athletes to have attitudes that promote injuries.

The coach has the opportunity to take a stand against what seems to be an insatiable appetite for violence in America. People love a female hockey player who knocks an opponent into the boards. The crowd cheers when a quarterback gets clotheslined and almost has his head ripped off. The coach can encourage young athletes to embrace the finer aspects of sports, not the cheap thrills of violence.

Coaches behave unprofessionally when they get hung up on the fantasy of professional sports and try to apply it to school-level teams. For example, one of the most dangerous sports techniques taught by some football coaches is spearing, a blocking and tackling technique that requires initial contact with the head. Because of modern hard plastic football helmets, the head can be used as a weapon to punish opponents, but spearing has resulted in an increase in serious neck injuries that often have tragic consequences. Although the governing bodies of football at all levels of play have rules prohibiting this technique, spearing is still taught by many coaches. It's important that parents support the teaching of basic sports fundamentals that promote sports safety rather than dangerous techniques designed to hurt an opponent.

The positive effects of sports should always outweigh the negative ones. A lifetime with a bad knee is a big price to pay for poor judgment by an over ambitious coach. Fortunately, serious injuries rarely happen in children's sports, because the vast majority of coaches are extremely competent and they take every precaution to insure the safety of your child.

Coaches sometimes adopt training methods and attitudes that are contrary to current medical knowledge. Every fall football players die from heat stroke, a condition in which the body loses control of the ability to regulate temperature. These deaths are tragic and completely unnecessary. Athletes should be encouraged (or even forced) to drink plenty of water when they engage in heavy exercise, particularly in hot and humid weather. It's surprising how many coaches are ignorant about the importance of fluids during exercise. Some coaches even withhold water from players, in the hope of "making them tough." Research by countless sports medicine scientists has shown conclusively that an adequate water intake is essential for keeping body temperature within normal ranges. The natural thirst of the athlete is not enough to accomplish this, since dehydration and rising body temperature will exceed the thirst for water. It's therefore important for athletes to drink more water than they feel they need. Athletes can easily learn to consume water during exercise—in fact, it will improve their performance.

What the Parent Can Do

Physical conditioning is one of the most important factors preventing athletic injuries. Parents can encourage their children to remain fit during the entire year, not just when the sport is in season. Frantic fitness programs two weeks before the season make the athlete a candidate for injury and, at the very least, result in poor performance. Many schools have rules against sports practices during the off-season. Although these rules were instituted to prevent overemphasis of sports, they often result in athletes being poorly prepared for the rigors of competitive athletics. It's up to parents to assume part of the responsibility for encouraging fitness in their children.

A physical conditioning program should continue throughout the year. Immediately after the season, emphasize well-rounded general conditioning. Encourage your child to systematically develop endurance, strength, power, flexibility, agility, and speed. Consistency is the key. The intensity doesn't have to be as severe as during the actual season. Young athletes should begin early to plan their training program and keep a written record of it. Help children to set attainable, short-term goals. For example, a young runner might move up to running six to ten miles a day within a year; a football player might have a goal of lifting a particular weight or performing a certain number of chin-ups. People always work harder when they have a realistic goal and can see their improvement. Parents can help their children set their goals and provide encouragement to attain them.

One of the most important things parents can do is help their child develop good posture. Poor posture is a cause of many injuries, particularly to the back. With good posture, the child should be able to remain standing or seated for a reasonably long period of time with little effort. Bones and their ligamentous attachments should be aligned so that the athlete needs little muscular exertion to maintain a particular body position. However, when the child assumes an inefficient body posture, his muscles o assist. These muscles can easily fatigue and stress the joints and ligaments of the spine that are so critical for maintaining painless postures. Although there are some bad postures due to structural and genetic abnormalities, most posture problems are due to bad habits learned in childhood.

Adolescent postures often reflect the way they feel about themselves psychologically. The athlete, after losing a game or making a mistake, might be slumped and dejected. His head is bowed and he walks with a slow shuffle—the classic "agony of defeat" posture. Children with negative attitudes about themselves may develop this type of drooped stance as a chronic habit. These slouching postures quickly fatigue and stress the supportive structures of the back and neck. This is another example of the importance of

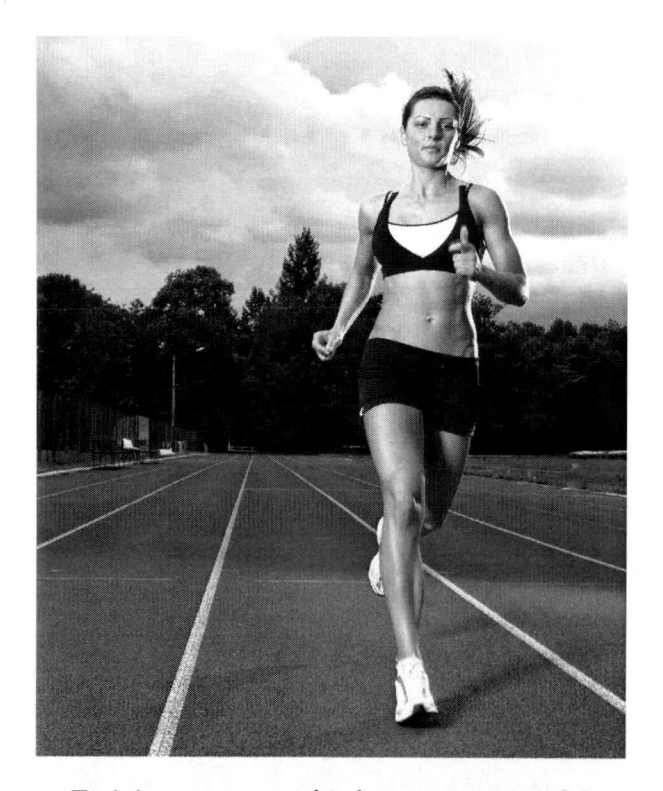

Training year-round is key to a successful physical conditioning program.

developing positive attitudes in children. Good self-image promotes emotional and physical well-being.

Coaches and parents should encourage prudent living habits. Growing children need adequate rest and a well-balanced diet. Unfortunately, our fast-food society makes empty-calorie snacks look very desirable. Children need to be educated about the need for proper nutrition and the hazards of drugs, smoking, and alcohol, and should receive this health education from an early age, both at home and at school. It will be valuable in confronting the social pressures most children are subjected to, particularly as teenagers. Our children are fat and getting fatter. Studies published in late 2002 showed that more than 15% of our school children are overweight—an increase of 30% in less than 10 years. Lack of exercise and poor diet account for much of this.

Good Equipment

Modern synthetics have revolutionized athletic equipment, from tennis racquets and skis to running surfaces and playing fields. Unfortunately, inferior equipment is often given to children under the guise of "junior models." Inadequate equipment may decrease performance or even cause injury. A loose-fitting football helmet may result in a head or neck injury. Ski bindings that don't release can result in a broken leg. A tennis racquet too large for a child may cause elbow or shoulder pain. Children must have good-quality equipment that fits properly.

Safety equipment should be mandatory. Children in sports like skateboarding, snow boarding, and skiing should wear a helmet.

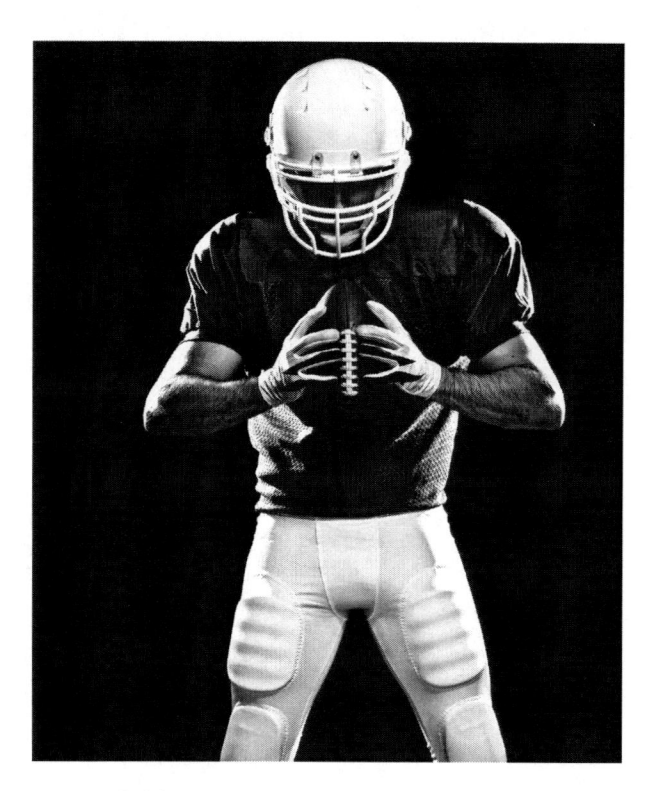

Children must have quality sporting equipment and clothing that fits properly.

Children should learn that they must always wear a life jacket when sailing, water skiing, or river rafting. Kids often tempt fate by acting foolhardy. Although this is part of growing up, they should use safety equipment for their own good.

Medical Supervision

Proper medical supervision of your child is in the hands of three people: the physician who assesses the child's suitability for sports and directly assumes responsibility for treatment of injuries; the athletic trainer who supervises rehabilitation of injuries; and the coach or personal trainer who directly supervises the health care of the child athlete on the field or in the gym. Each has definite responsibilities. In cases where money is a problem, parents

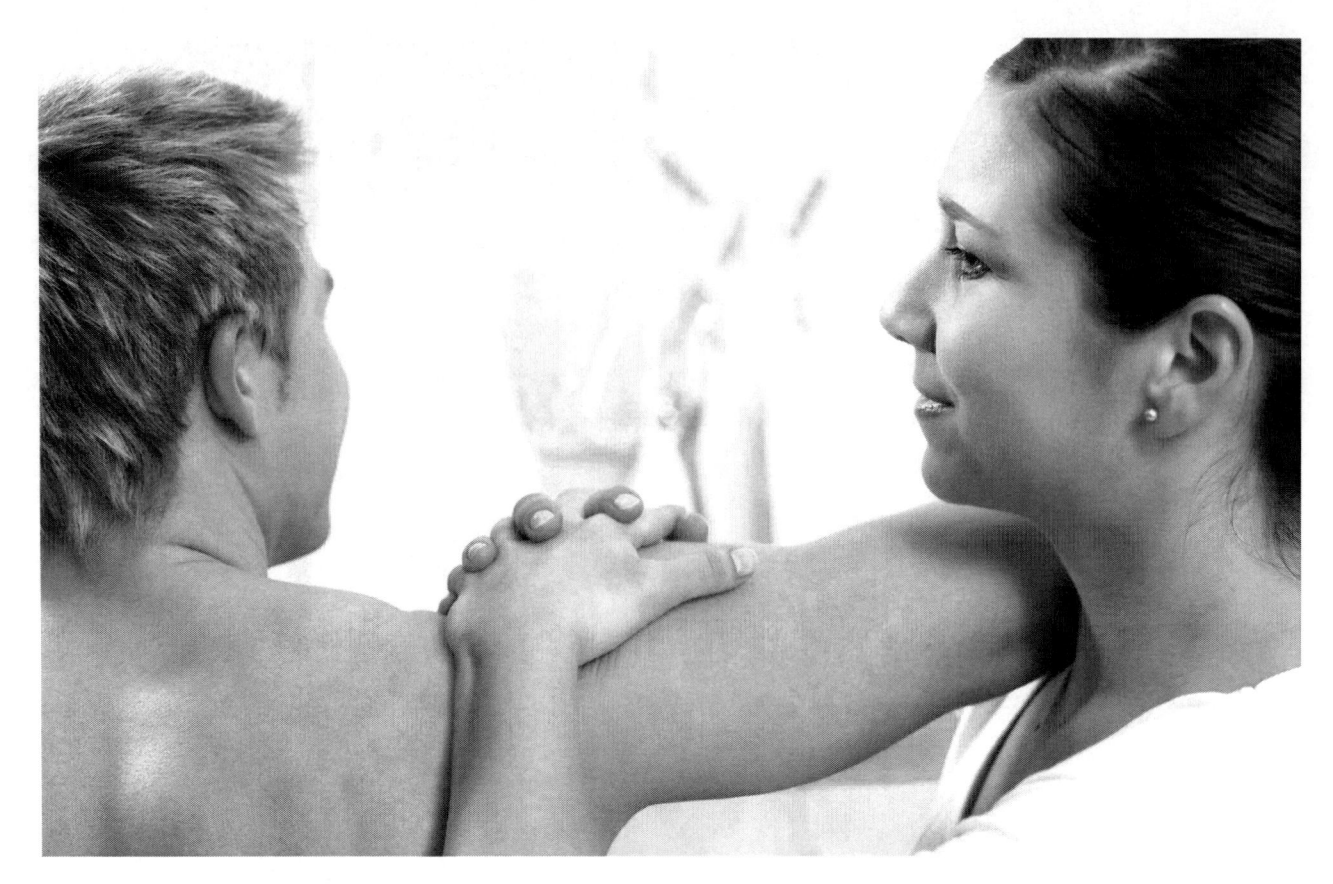

Sports physicians can determine when an athlete should play or rest.

will have to assume the first-aid responsibilities that should ideally be the doctor's.

Child athletes should get regular physical examinations by a physician. Ideally, the physician should have a good knowledge of growth and development and a familiarity with sports medicine. An orthopedic specialist should evaluate injuries involving bones and joints, particularly in bone growth centers. Team doctors are usually the best for treating athletic injuries, since most of them have had a lot of experience. They often have the best judgment on when athletes should play and when they should rest.

The duties of the children's sports physician include:

• To determine if the child has the physical maturity to safely participate in a sport.

• To restrict a child from a sport if he or she has medical problems.

• To recommend to children with medical problems alternative sports and physical activities appropriate for their condition.

• To obtain prompt treatment of conditions encountered in the health examination.

A physician should be present during any athletic contest that involves a risk of serious injury. Sports that particularly need direct medical supervision are boys' football and wrestling, and girls' and boys' basketball. If possible, a physician should be on call for football practices, as most injuries occur during training and practice sessions. Ideally, one physician should be involved in an organization's entire athletic program, to provide a consistency of health care and better readiness for emergencies. The physician should always have emergency equipment available.

A surprising number of athletic teams, particularly at the elementary school and junior high levels, have no medical supervision at all. The community should strive to improve the health care in sports at all levels. At the very least, qualified athletic trainers should be available to help fill the void. If no trainer is available, then the coaches should have a good knowledge of first aid and emergency procedures.

When to Call the Doctor

Children get all kinds of bumps and bruises during the course of organized athletics and impromptu sports and games, . If you ran to your doctor every time this happened, you would quickly drain the time and resources of you and your physician.

Most minor injuries to muscles and joints don't require medical examination. The orthopedic specialists whom I consulted indicated that people should "wait and see" before consulting a physician for most muscle and joint injuries. It's difficult to list hard and fast rules for separating serious from relatively benign athletic injuries, but there are some general guidelines:

• The proper way to treat tennis elbow, sore muscles, Achilles tendon pains, and other overuse injuries is to gradually progress from initial rest to stretching and then to systematic strengthening. However, if the pain from an overuse injury does not disappear after several weeks, take your child to a physician.

• Head and eye injuries require immediate medical attention; "traumatic" injuries, caused by sudden blows or an overwhelming force, that will usually result in swelling-particularly to such joints as the ankle and knee; injuries involving damage to the ligaments, which hold bones together; injuries involving broken bones; and internally related disorders such as chest pains, fainting, and intolerance to heat. Unless the injury is obviously minor, get your child to a doctor as quickly as possible. Be careful not to underestimate the seriousness of an injury.

• Teach children to "listen" to their bodies. If the pain from an injury is beyond tolerance, get medical attention quickly. But if the pain is only a spasm or cramp from overexertion, there is very little a doctor can do. Think of how the injury happened: a back injury sustained when five defensive players stomped on your child's spine may call for an X-ray; a backache caused by a hefty swing through a "gopher" pitch may not.

Common Injuries and Disabilities in Children's Sports

Specific treatment of athletic injuries in children's athletics is beyond the scope of this book. However, it's important that you know the general principles involved in sports injuries and disabilities commonly experienced by children.

Injuries to Joints and Muscles

Joint and muscle injuries are common in children's sports, but are usually relatively benign if cared for properly. In general, the immediate care of these injuries involves immobilization, ice, elevation, and compression.

Very often after a child sustains an injury such as a pulled muscle, sprained ankle, or twisted knee, function appears to be almost normal. The tendency is often to "run it off." Because the muscle is warm and initial swelling is minimal, a child can easily underestimate the seriousness an injury. Continued playing with an injury is only going to make things worse and delay recovery. It's important that the injured area be iced, immobilized, elevated, and rested.. Although the athlete may want to maintain motion in the joint, he or she should try to do so without putting too much weight on it.

Immediate Treatment

One of the best things an athlete can do to speed recovery from an injury is to ice the area. Ice will numb the injured area and block much of the pain by slowing down the activity of the nerves that send pain sensations. A good ice treatment will relax the injured area and reduce the muscle spasms that may occur, and at the same time increase the blood flow deep in the tissue without causing swelling.

Cryokinetics, which entails moving an injured area after an initial cooling with ice, has brought important breakthroughs in the treatment of athletic injuries. Until recently, the immediate treatment of an injury was limited to immobilization followed by heat treatment and massage. Cryokinetics requires the athlete to take the weight off the injured area to a certain extent, but also involves an attempt to regain and maintain the area's full range of motion. A sprained ankle, for instance, would be treated by applying an ice pack, wrapping the ankle in an elastic bandage, and elevating the foot. Then, the injured athlete would try to move his foot forward and backward, and downward and upward. Immobilization of the ankle is followed by an attempt to regain the full range of foot motion.

An injured child can quickly recover full range of motion in the injured area and normal use of his body through continued ice therapy. Also, continued ice treatment can prevent much of the deconditioning that often results from an injury, since the therapy will reduce pain and muscle spasms. Ice treatment, because it does not eliminate all pain sensations, keeps you from overdoing it and possibly making the injury worse.

The most common types of ice treatment are the ice massage, the ice bath, and the ice pack. The ice massage is very effective for cooling a particular spot. Fill a paper cup with water and freeze it. When the ice is formed, peel away the upper half of the cup and hold the ice by the lower half of the cup. Using a circular motion, massage the injured area for seven to ten minutes, or until numbness sets in. You can avoid numbing your fingers by placing a tongue depressor in the cup of water before making the ice. This will create a large frozen lollipop with a convenient handle. A word of caution: Never use dry ice.

An ice pack is valuable for immediate treatment of muscle and joint injuries. Take a wet towel and place a layer of crushed ice on it, then wrap or place the towel directly on the injury. Another method of ice packing involves placing a plastic bag filled with ice directly on the injury. However, this kind of ice pack is less effective because the ice is often unevenly distributed. Commercially available ice packs can be carried in your athletic bag until needed. Breaking a container inside the pack activates a chemical reaction that creates a cold ice pack that lasts for 20 to 30 minutes. Immersion in ice water can be effective for injuries to the ankles, hands, feet, elbows, and sometimes knees. You can also use the ice bath during the later stages of injury rehabilitation, when it's no longer necessary to elevate the injured part. Add about two-dozen ice cubes to a sink or basin filled with cold water. Immerse the injured area in the ice water and leave it there. If you are only able to tolerate a few minutes, take the injured part out of the water for about a minute, and then reimmerse it for seven to eight minutes. Keeping an injured area in the ice water for more than ten minutes will do little good. In fact, you risk developing frostbite by immersing an injury for too long.

After the swelling of an injured area has subsided, heat can be used to increase circulation and relax the muscles. Since effective healing cannot progress until swelling decreases, heat should not be used sooner than 48 to 72 hours after a muscle or joint injury has been sustained. Premature heat therapy may actually increase swelling and retard the healing process. This is especially true in injuries that entail muscle pulls and joint damage, which are usually accompanied by damage to the blood vessels.

Heat can be administered in several different ways. The hot bath, or whirlpool, is probably the easiest. Water temperature should be kept between 90' and 112° Fahrenheit, with 105° being comfortable for most people. Never allow your child to use a hot whirlpool bath if he or she has lost the tactile sense; in this kind of injury, the body may be more susceptible to bums. Other kinds of heat treatment include hot water bottles, heating pads, L packs (silicone-filled canvas bags heated in water), and heat lamps.

Rehabilitation

Rehabilitating muscle and joint injuries is critical. After an injury, the body attempts to protect itself by producing muscle spasms and adhesions in joints that restrict motion. Psychologically, the natural tendency is to baby the injury in an attempt to keep it from getting worse.

I know of many athletes who fail to restore normal function after an injury, and they never seem to get any better. Athletes must work hard to restore as much strength, flexibility, and endurance as possible. Start gradually and systematically increase the intensity of rehabilitation exercises until normal function is restored.

An injured child should try to rehabilitate the injury as much as possible before returning to full sports participation. The physician should determine when to return to practice when the injury is serious. Rest from sports is often necessary for optimal healing; an injured part of the body that's not completely healed is extremely vulnerable to reinjury. There are some general principles you can follow to help your child decide when to return to sports:

• The child should not return to sports until the injured area is completely restored to its full range of motion—both actively and passively. Simply recovering the ability to move the knee, shoulder, or elbow in a non-active situation is not enough rehabilitation. The body must be able to withstand the rigors of sports as well as it did before the injury.

• Regain full strength and power before returning to active sports. Compare the injured side with the uninjured side to see if size and strength are equal. If not, more rehabilitation of the injury is necessary before resuming play.

• Restore full range of motion before returning to sports. All compensating motions, such as limping and favoring an injured area, should be eliminated. After a lower body injury, for instance, rehabilitation is not complete unless you can run forward, backward, and laterally. You must also recover your ability to start and stop quickly.

• The injured athlete should be relatively free of pain. Some pain is a natural part of sports; the old football maxim, "You've got to play with small hurts," is true. However, the rehabilitation process is not yet complete if the pain is intolerable.

Overuse Injuries

Many young athletes can become over-motivated—they train like they're trying to make the Olympic team in a month. Overuse injuries occur when athletes train beyond the tolerance of their bodies. Examples include shin splints, sore Achilles tendons, and tennis elbow. These injuries result from overworking relatively weak areas and from improper sports techniques. Modem training methods increase overuse injuries. It's not uncommon for young swimmers to put in 10,000 meters per day, or for young distance runners to cover 75 miles a week. These brutal training programs do produce results. Competitive records by young athletes continue to fall. However, the young athlete is often pushed too far, too fast. And often there is inadequate preparation or buildup for these difficult exercise programs. Overuse injuries can be tricky to deal with, particularly because the ultimate responsibility for rehabilitation lies with the athlete. Sometimes athletes must rest in order to heal and improve performance.

Often associated with the overuse injury is the overtraining syndrome. This condition is particularly prevalent in highly motivated athletes. The overtrained athlete feels sluggish, tired, sore, and may lack enthusiasm. Often he or she will perform well during practice but blow it during competition. Many coaches would call this the "choke" syndrome.

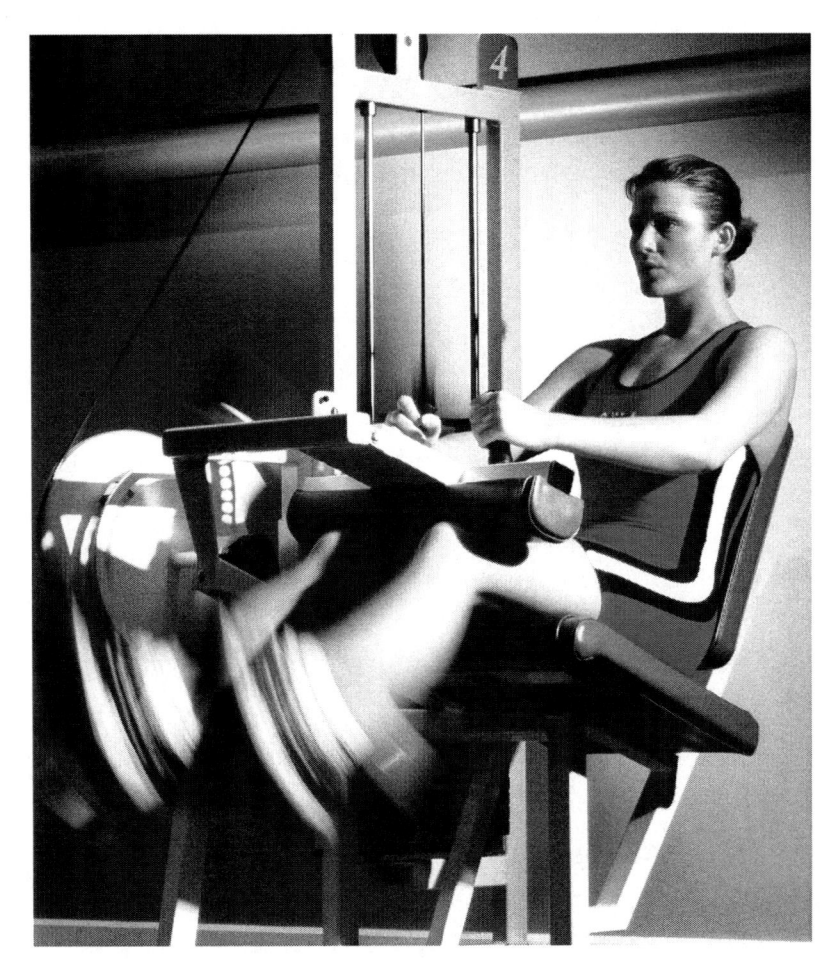

The use of exercise equipment can help restore normal function and range of motion after an injury.

However, sports scientists have recently shown that overtraining is at least partially due to lack of an important muscle fuel, glycogen. Glycogen, the complex carbohydrate that is so important for muscular exercise, is depleted by overtraining. When muscles run low on this fuel, they ache and don't perform as well. Overtraining is related to overuse injuries—when an athlete is fatigued and run down, injury is just around the corner. Other factors, such as depressed testosterone and glutamine levels may also contribute to the symptoms of overtraining.

Rest is very important for the overtrained athlete. Rest is the only thing that can break the vicious cycle—the hard training athlete does poorly in competition, so he trains even harder. The harder he trains, the more he depletes his muscle fuel supplies. Competitive performances keep getting worse. The best thing for the overtrained athlete is to take a few days off and to check the carbohydrate content of his diet. Athletes involved in vigorous training should include large amounts of carbohydrates in his diet to maximize muscle fuel stores.

Imbalance Injuries

Poor posture, training that overdevelops some muscle groups at the expense of others, and anatomical weaknesses promote imbalance injuries. Normal movements usually don't involve undue risk of injury. But sports, by

ATHLETIC INJURIES | **117**

their very nature, require stretching a little further or trying a little harder. When you add such factors as fatigue, anxiety, anger, poor body mechanics, and bad luck, weak links in the body's structure can be overwhelmed—injury may be inevitable.

Muscle imbalances often cause injuries. Some people develop the muscles on the front of the thigh (quadriceps), for example, without also developing the muscles on the back of the thigh (hamstrings). This causes an imbalance that may result in hamstring pulls. Back pains are also caused by poor muscle fitness and imbalances. Back trouble is usually accompanied by unfit abdominal, back, and leg muscles, and inflexible hamstring and back muscles.

The upright posture has resulted in many aches and pains that four-legged animals don't have. Many children have minor anatomical imbalances that throw their bodies out of balance and increase the risk of injury. For instance, having one leg longer than the other can cause pain in the back, knees, or hips.

Growth Plate Injuries

The growth plate, or epiphyseal plate, is the portion of the bone where growth occurs. When full growth is complete, this area fuses and the growth plate disappears. Bone growth at the epiphyseal plate depends upon its blood supply; injury interferes with blood supply and can impair growth.

Sports and exercise can affect bone growth in different ways. The mild stress of active play and sports stimulates bone strength and resiliency, because bones adapt to the stresses and strains placed upon them. Bones of active athletes have a larger diameter and a larger marrow cavity (the portion of bones where red blood cells are produced). However, severe stress can inflame bone and cause an interruption of normal bone growth.

Growth plate injuries in children's sport include separation of growth plate; a bone break or fracture that goes through the growth plate; and crush injuries to the growth plate. These injuries can occur by sudden contact, as when a child tries to break a fall with outstretched arms, or from violent twisting motions such as might occur during skiing. Growth plate injuries can also occur more subtly from such repeated movement as throwing or running. The more subtle growth plate injuries can be classified as part of the overuse syndrome, and can be difficult to diagnose. So-called sprains around joints such as the fingers, ankles, elbows, knees, or shoulders may really be growth plate injuries. Proper diagnosis often requires the advice of an orthopedic specialist. Chronic pain may be a sign of growth plate injury, and should be investigated.

Fortunately, growth plate injuries are fairly uncommon, accounting for only six percent of all injuries in children's athletics. Because children have relatively weak muscles and low body weight, they do not often develop the force that causes these injuries. However, there are certain children who are at increased risk. Overweight children, for example, can create forces strong enough to cause growth plate injury. In rapidly growing children, muscle development can lag and leave bones, joints, and growth plates more vulnerable to injury. And after an illness or injury, muscles may be deconditioned to such an extent that growth plates are more susceptible to harm. Children should build themselves up after a period of deconditioning before resuming active athletics.

Throwing sports, such as pitching or javelin throwing, may place an unusual strain on bone growth centers. These conditions, known by such names as little league shoulder, javelin elbow, or little league elbow, seem to be caused by too much throwing and, to a certain extent, poor technique. They have resulted in a great deal of misunderstanding and, in some circles, a bad reputation for Little League baseball.

The Little League has rules which limit the amount of a player's pitching. These limits are well within the bounds of safety. Unfortunately, children usually practice pitching on their own, in addition to official practice. It's the extra strain of the outside practice that usually causes the problems.

The method of delivery is an important factor in throwing injuries. There were many more injuries when pitchers used a sidearm delivery as opposed to a throw that comes right over the top. While this remains controversial, it is certain that the coach should limit or stop athletes from throwing if they have arm pain. A player's continued participation when he has a throwing injury could lead to problems later in life, and perhaps hamper further athletic development.

Javelin throwing can easily result in growth plate injuries in children. Because of the weight of the implement, errors in throwing technique can have a severe effect on bone growth centers. Children should not throw the javelin until they are skeletally mature, usually at sixteen to eighteen years. The natural tendency of beginning throwers is to use a sidearm motion, which disposes them to injury. Proper technique requires expert coaching, which is rarely available to young adolescents.

Osgood-Schlatter Disease

The term Osgood-Schlatter disease refers to an overuse injury, not an actual disease. Adolescents often experience pain, swelling, and tenderness in the area just below the kneecap, where the patella ligament connects to the bony growth on the center of the upper part of the tibia (the large bone of your lower leg). This condition is commonly called Osgood-Schlatter disease, and it is caused by repeated small tears at the point where the ligament connects to the bone. Osgood-Schlatter usually afflicts girls between eight and thirteen years and boys between ten and fifteen years, although boys are about three times more susceptible than girls. The condition will result in pain during such activities as kneeling, direct contact with objects, running, and climbing. It can be curbed through rest and restriction from activities, although it will probably not disappear completely until after the child is fully grown. Consult a physician if you suspect the child has this problem.

Mononucleosis

Infectious mononucleosis is characterized by such cold-like symptoms as sore throat, fever, enlarged lymph nodes in the neck, and general fatigue. It is caused by the Epstein-Barr virus that's carried in the throat and bloodstream. Many people have developed immunity to mononucleosis by producing an antibody to the disease. Those who don't produce the antibody are susceptible to the illness.

The symptoms of mononucleosis usually last 14 to 21 days. The disease is often accompanied by an enlarged spleen, the size of which is an important consideration when determining if an athlete is ready to return to play. The spleen serves as a reservoir and cleanser of the blood; if it is enlarged, it can easily be ruptured in contact sports. An athlete with mononucleosis and an enlarged spleen should be examined and cleared by a physician. Most physicians recommend a delay of three to four weeks after the disappearance of symptoms before returning to sports such as football and basketball.

Preventing mononucleosis is often difficult. It can be transmitted by kissing or drinking from a contaminated cup or pop bottle. Perhaps you can encourage your child not to date until thirty years of age and, after that, to keep any fooling around to a minimum.

Asthma

Asthma is a breathing disorder characterized by choking, shortness of breath, tightness in the chest, increased mucus production, and fatigue. There are over 1.5 million asthmatic children in the United States, most of whom tend to shun sports and vigorous physical activity. This is understandable, because exercise is one of the prime precipitators of asthma attacks. Many parents, coaches, school administrators, and even physicians advise asthmatics not to take part in sports and normal physical education. However, advances in medicine have enabled asthmatics to excel at vigorous sports, even to the point of winning Olympic medals.

Research has shown two factors to be important in preventing asthmatic attacks during and following exercise: medication and environment. Modern medications enable asthmatics to participate in even the most vigorous sports by either preventing exercise-induced asthma or reducing its effects once they have occurred. If you suspect your child has asthma, see a physician; in most instances, he or she can lead a normal life.

Environmental factors should be considered in the exercise program of the asthmatic. Exercise should be modified or curtailed when the child is too tired or under excessive emotional stress, on cold, foggy, or humid days, and on days when there is a high smog level. Swimming in cold pools can also cause an asthma attack. Under adverse environmental conditions, exercise bouts should be kept short—less than three minutes at a time. However, the exercise levels should be adjusted to individual tolerance.

Instant Replay

- Parents, coaches, and trainers should help their child keep athletics and athletic injuries in perspective. When an injured young athlete plays with the injury or fails to fully rehabilitate it, he may be risking a lifetime of discomfort and lack of function.

- Prevent injuries with proper coaching, good equipment, proper medical supervision, and physical conditioning.

- The immediate care of muscle and joint injuries includes immobilization, elevation, ice, and compression. Rehabilitation of these injuries should include restoration of range of motion, strength, and endurance.

- An athlete with a muscle or joint injury should not return to normal athletic play until full strength, power, and range of motion is restored. Movement should be normal without compensating movements such as limping. The child should be relatively pain free.

- Overuse and overtraining injuries are often caused by doing too much, too soon. Rest is important in overuse conditions, and often produces better performance than heavy training.

- Imbalance injuries can produce pains in the knees, hips, and back. They are caused by such factors as poor posture, imbalanced muscle groups, or anatomical abnormalities.

- Growth plate injuries are of great concern in children's sports. They can be caused by sudden traumatic injuries in sports like skiing or football, or by overuse in throwing sports or running.

- Asthmatic children can participate in sports if they receive the proper medication and are afforded individual consideration during adverse environmental, physical, or emotional conditions.

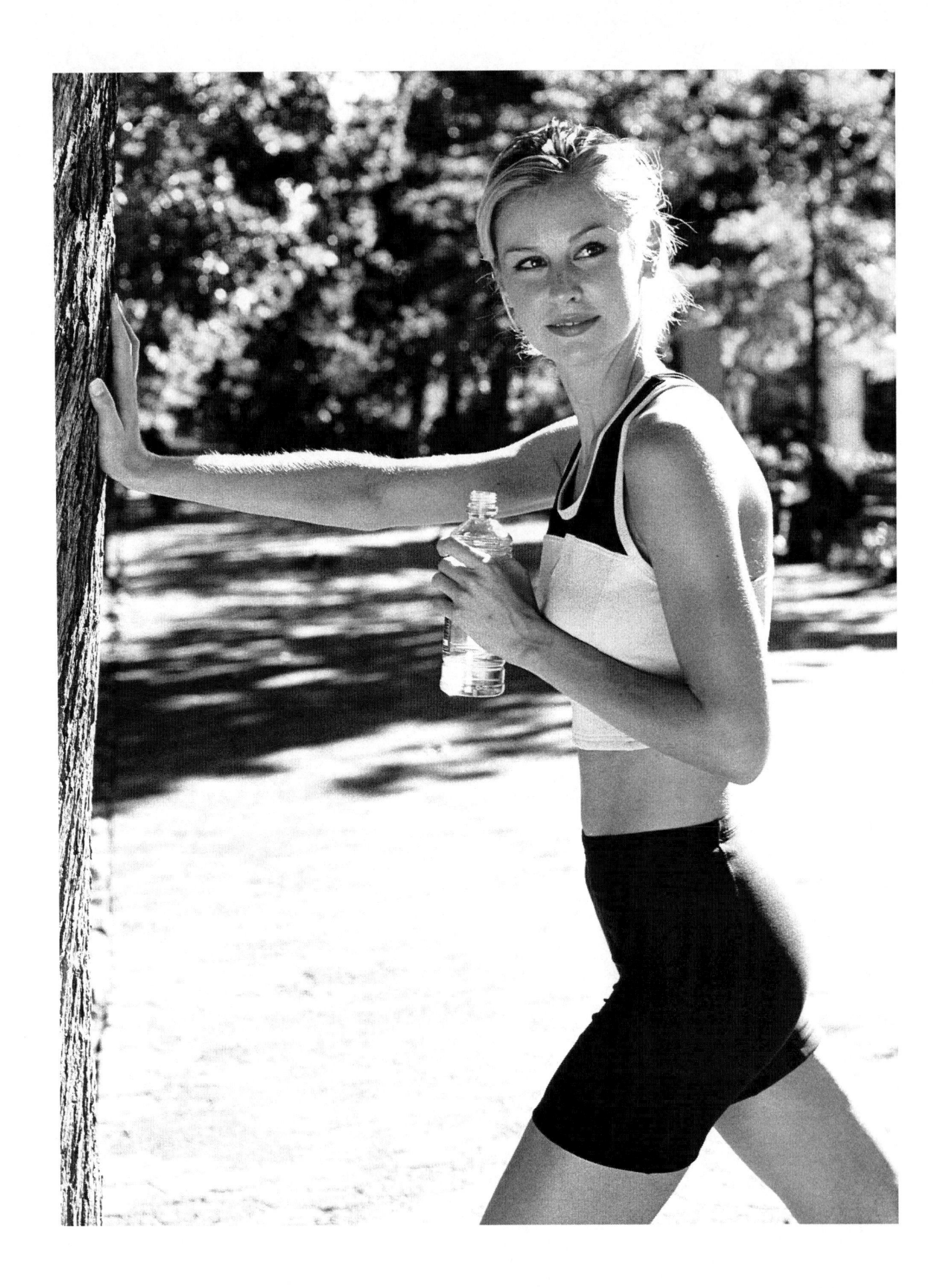

Developing an Active Lifestyle

"The sweat and sacrifice of today will produce the memories of tomorrow." So reads a sign in the office of a local football coach. In some ways, that inspirational slogan summarizes much that is right and much that is wrong with athletics in this country. The competitive sports of youth do indeed produce wonderful memories for many. Friendships acquired in childhood sports can last a lifetime, and the former athlete has the satisfaction of having belonged to something that represented accomplishment, excellence, enthusiasm, and hope.

However, sports should provide more than just memories. Sports and physical activity should be integrated into everyone's lifestyle, beyond senior high school. An ex-athlete who dwells on the past may be living an illusion—and is probably sedentary as well. I find it very disturbing that the extent of the athletic experience for many modern sports people is vicarious participation. The lives of these 50-yard-line athletes ebb and flow with the fortunes of a few highly conditioned superstars. These same spectators who holler so loudly when a pro player makes a mistake couldn't run a mile themselves without risking exhaustion or heart attack.

Sports during youth should educate children for the future. Physical activity should become a positive habit that can be integrated into adult living patterns. If the sum total of the worth of athletics is to provide memories for sedentary adults, then school districts can save themselves a lot of money by eliminating the sports program.

Sports and physical activity can be among the most important experiences of children. They can and should provide tools to promote health and vitality for a lifetime, along with a variety of recreational outlets that increase enjoyment and produce personal satisfaction.

Sports, Exercise, and Health

Throughout the book I've described specific exercise programs for children from infancy through adolescence. The aim of these programs is to improve organic vigor directly through such activities as running, swimming, and hiking, or to develop fitness indirectly by teaching basic movement skills and sports fundamentals. From the standpoint of health, an exercise program should fulfill several requirements: it should develop at least a minimum level of cardiovascular

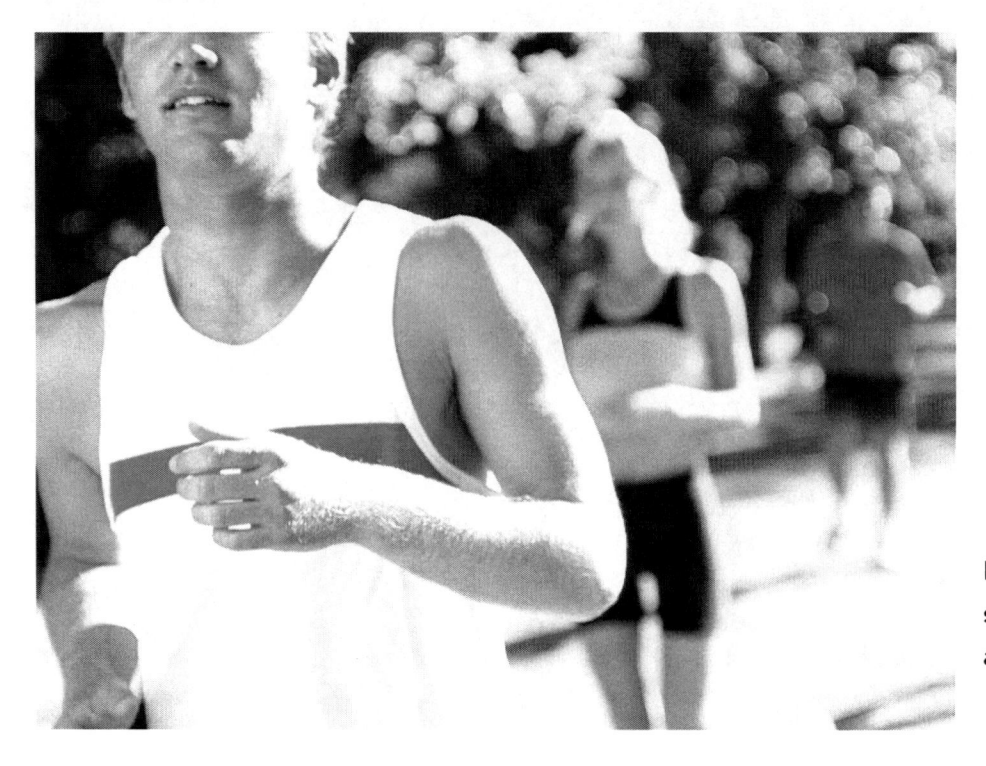

Endurance exercise should be the core of any fitness program.

fitness; it should develop and maintain adequate muscle strength and flexibility; it should help control body fat.

Cardiovascular Fitness

Endurance exercise, sometimes called aerobics, promotes cardiovascular health and should be at the core of any fitness program. Cardiovascular exercise should be practiced throughout a lifetime. Here are the basics of a minimum cardiovascular exercise program:

• It should be an aerobic exercise—one that uses large-muscle groups rhythmically and continuously for a long period of time.

• It should be practiced three to five times a week.

• Each training session should be at least 20 to 30 minutes long.

• The level of exercise should exceed 60 to 85 percent of maximum capacity. The heart rate can be used as a guide to find the proper exercise intensity.

In 1996, the Surgeon General of the United States—based on the advice of exercise experts— recommended that Americans exercise moderately for 30 minutes a day. They made a distinction between fitness and exercise. While the recommendation recognized the value of exercising more than 30 minutes a day, they set that level as the minimum goal for the average person. That isn't much, but 50% of American don't do that much. Only 12% exercise intensely enough to satisfy the recommendations for developing fitness as described above.

Muscle Strength and Flexibility

Muscle strength and flexibility are important for preventing aches and pains in areas such as the back, neck, and shoulders. Strength and flexibility can be developed directly through specific exercises, or indirectly through participation in a variety of sports.

Controlling Body Fat

The exercise program should help control body fat. A lifelong weight control program should be instituted during childhood and adolescence. Research studies have shown that an obese teenager has an 85% chance of becoming an obese adult. Childhood obesity is associated with low self-esteem, social isolation, and feelings of rejection and depression. The negative psychological effects of excess body fat can spill over into academic, social, and physical pursuits. Unfortunately, in 2002, more than 15% of our children are classified as overweight.

Obesity during childhood and adolescence is caused by a caloric intake that is higher than necessary for the body's energy needs and expenditures. Overeating is not always the primary cause. Obese children are almost always physically inactive, and even when they do play games, they tend to move a lot less than leaner kids. Add to this, the problems associated with fast food diets high in simple sugars and saturated fats.

Effective weight control is especially important during a child's growing years, when fat cells can increase in number. In adults, fat cells increase only in size. Dieting does not decrease fat cell number, only fat cell size. Thus, an overeating or inactive child will develop fat cells that can never be lost, and this will create a hopelessly obese adult. Unless weight control begins during childhood, to the child will be a slave to a lifetime of crash diets and rapid weight gains.

Many overweight children try drastic short-term weight control programs that usually fail. Fasting is extremely popular and also extremely ineffective. Even though fasting people lose body weight, much of it is muscle tissue. This has two effects: first, these crash diets make people look ghastly because of the loss of muscle tone; second, the loss of muscle tissue decreases the metabolic rate, making the newly lost weight difficult to keep off. Other short-term programs that involve "fat farms," hormone therapy using thyroid hormone and human chorionic gonadotropin, weight loss drugs, and unbalanced diets tend to be ineffective, ill-advised, and potentially dangerous.

Long-term management of obesity is the only answer. Children must undertake a program of behavior modification that involves caloric restriction, a balanced diet, exercise, and sports. Children must be supported psychologically, since obesity is very often caused by emotional problems. Parents should be understanding; rather than criticizing an overweight child, take steps to aid in weight control. Some suggestions are:

• Serve small portions at mealtime. Overeating is often learned at the dinner table. Some families eat the amount served, even if it is too much. Smaller portions mean fewer calories. Teach children that eating more calories causes weight gain.

- Serve foods lower in calories. Try to serve more fish and poultry—these foods are lower in calories than beef. Make sure to serve vegetables, which add bulk to the meal while adding few calories. Try to avoid butter and sour cream when serving bread and potatoes.

- Use low-fat or non-fat milk. Children can quickly develop a taste for these products if they stop drinking whole milk. Young children should not drink non-fat milk because they need the milk fat to help them develop their nervous systems.

- Get rid of high-calorie desserts and junk food. For dessert, try fresh fruit. If you keep junk foods out of the house, there's less temptation. If you don't buy it, you can't eat it.

- Eat regular meals and discourage snacking. Children who skip breakfast often snack on high-calorie junk foods and get fat.

- Exercise as a family. Remember that children learn by example. Go for a walk after dinner, run as a family on weekends, or go on sports vacations. Children raised in an activity-oriented environment will be more likely to carry over exercise habits into adulthood.

Developing Skills in Lifetime Sports

Lifetime sports are activities that can be continued into adulthood. Although school sports are worthwhile for their own sake, they often have very little carryover after graduation. Couldn't you just hear a bunch of people talking at a cocktail party—"Hey, Sally, why don't we get a bunch of couples together and play tackle football and then wrestle down at the gym."

Although school sports can develop high levels of fitness and psychological traits helpful to the adult, they can also produce a recreationally bankrupt athlete. School athletics are no substitute for leisure-time activities that can be enjoyed for a lifetime.

Water Sports

Every child should learn to swim for self-preservation. The Red Cross has determined that if you haven't learned to swim by the time you're fifteen, chances are you never will. Even infants can learn to become familiar with the water and comfortable in it. If children learn to swim at an early age, they will never develop irrational fears of the water; they'll also learn their capabilities and limitations in the water.

Water sports can provide enjoyment for a lifetime. Teach children basic swimming skills as early as possible. Stress safety. Water sports are also particularly suited to family participation.

Although you can teach your child to swim yourself, enrollment in a swim school might work out better, because trained instructors are usually more effective in teaching swimming. Swimming should always be a positive experience. The worst thing you can do is to throw a kid in the water and let him "sink or swim." That looks like a great technique in macho western movies, but in reality it may cause children to fear water and shun swimming.

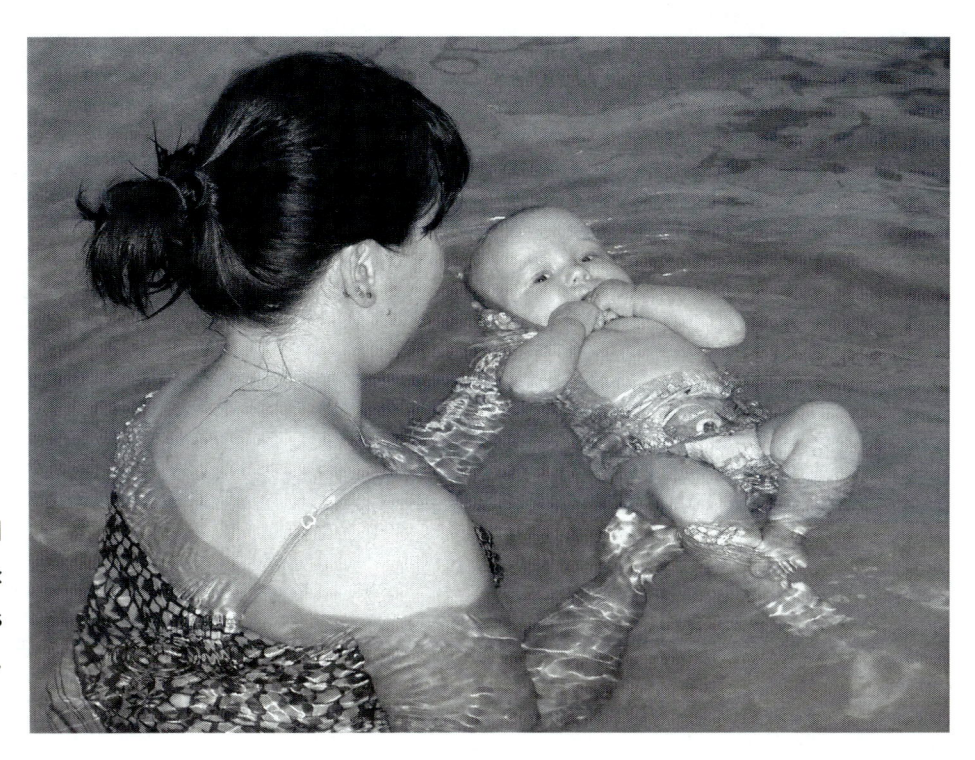

Children should be taught basic swimming skills as early as possible.

Early swimming lessons include activities that help children become comfortable in the water, like having the child put his face in the water and blow bubbles. Instructors will typically introduce games that teach floating, kicking, and beginning arm movements. With young children, instructors will often ask a parent to participate in the lessons—this reassures the child and reduces anxiety. Gradually, the lessons include and eventually introduce advanced techniques, such as diving.

Diving is a great activity for school-age children. This sport helps develop kinesthetic perception, the ability to feel the body position in a three-dimensional space. I recommend enrolling a child for diving lessons under the direction of a qualified teacher. You can learn about diving lessons from your local recreation department, YMCA, or after-school sports program.

Children can learn other water sports and activities after they learn to swim. The ocean can be a playground for children and adults alike. Body and board surfing are popular on both the east and west coasts, where nature has provided a natural roller coaster to play on. Inlanders in Arizona recently developed an artificial wave machine that simulates the ocean. Children should be fairly comfortable in water before attempting ocean sports, and should understand the dangers of rip tides and undertows before venturing into the surf. Above all, they should never go into the ocean alone. Although there is little danger of becoming a late-morning brunch for a great white shark, swimmers should always be wary in the ocean. People are the reverse of the proverbial "fish out of water" when they venture into the sea.

You must have training and certification for scuba diving before you can buy equipment.

DEVELOPING AN ACTIVE LIFESTYLE

Try introducing this sport via snorkeling or breath-hold diving. Scuba diving is safe when the diver receives proper training. Diving allows you to see some of the most incredible sights on earth, and can be a welcome addition to the active lifestyle.

Boating is a great family activity and lifetime sport. Whether you're out in a rowboat or a jet boat with a 450 Oldsmobile engine, boating can be a great way to spend a summer's day. You don't have to have a lot of money. Owning a boat can be a budget-buster, but you can rent one or join a cooperative boat club. Children usually love boating. Make sure you stress safety—always insist on life jackets and proper boating techniques. Children learn by example, and the habits of a safety-conscious adult will rub off.

Children love to water ski. They can learn this activity at about six or eight years of age. It's best to start kids off on two skis. Someone can hold the child steady in the water before starting on the first few runs. After a few tries, most kids will pop right up and put the adults to shame. Although water skiing can be a frightfully expensive sport, boats can be rented at most resorts at reasonable rates. If your family has never water skied, search out a family that does. Boat owners are always looking around for someone to share the fun.

River rafting is a new national craze. All your family needs to do it is a large raft or canoe and a river or lake. Many commercial organizations exist on major rivers across the country to guide you on river raft vacations. These rivers range from calm bodies of water

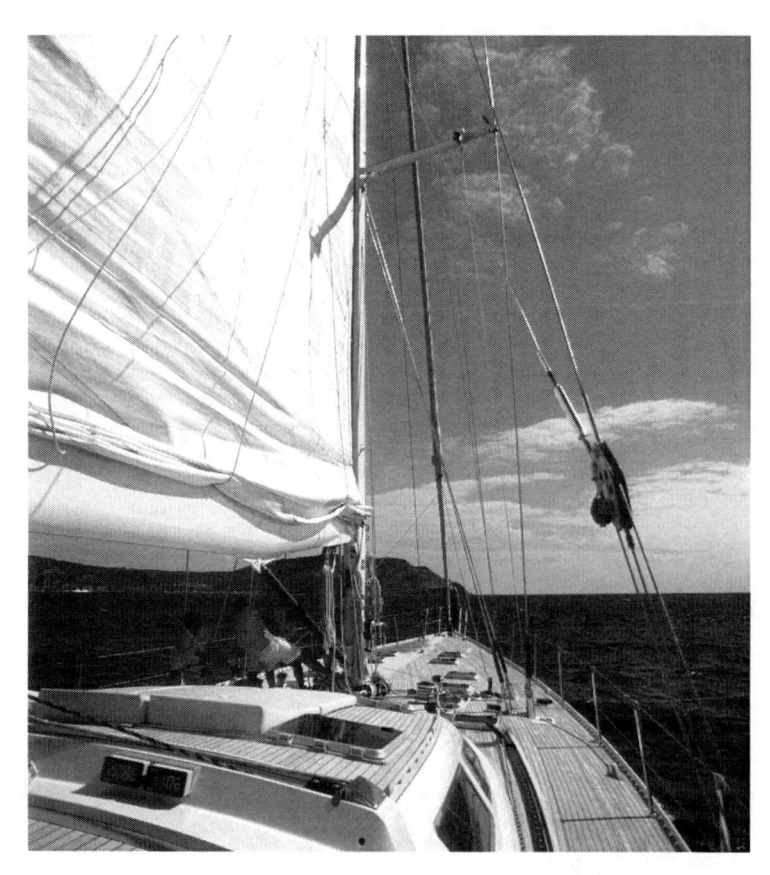

Boating: a great family activity and a lifetime sport.

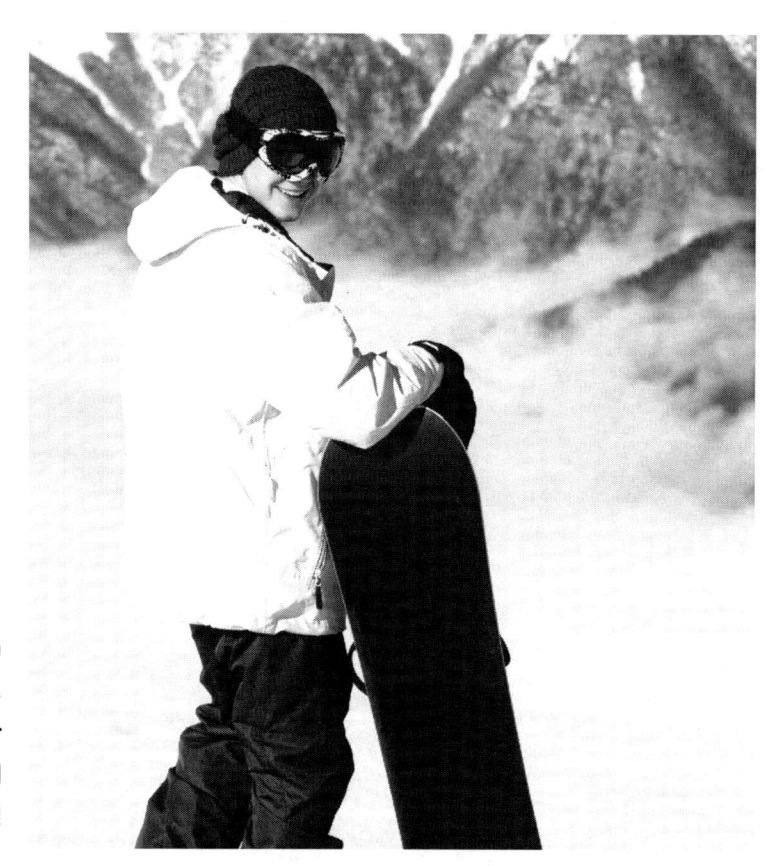

Almost all children love winter sports. Learning to ski or showboard should be fun!

that provide a leisurely sojourn down the waterway to hair-raising trips down the Colorado or Snake Rivers. Children should be introduced to this sport gently and gradually. Families are better off going on a guided trip before venturing off on their own.

Winter Sports

Snow sports are very popular with children and are good family recreation. Snow play is a natural for young children. Snowball fights, sledding, and tobogganing are a good introduction to winter sports. Remember, children cannot regulate their body temperature as well as adults can, so they should be adequately protected against the cold.

Snow Skiing

Skiing and snowboarding are extremely popular in the United States, Canada, and Europe. Children can put on a pair of skis soon after they learn to walk—at about one and a half to two years old. However, children won't learn real ski techniques until they're five or six. I think enjoyment should be the most important consideration with young kids. They can't be pushed to like the sport, and they certainly don't care if their technique is perfect. Treat each child as an individual—where one child may want to ski with Mommy and Daddy at three years, another may show no interest until later. Practice the sport in an atmosphere of fun and the child will want to participate. You won't have to push him.

DEVELOPING AN ACTIVE LIFESTYLE | **129**

Two of the most important considerations for the young skier are physical comfort and safety:

• Purchase the best possible equipment you can afford, but since equipment hunting for children can be mind boggling, learn as much as possible before making any decisions. Shop around and consult magazines such as Ski for information on the latest in ski equipment.

Stylish name brands are not always the way to go. Recently, I saw a skimpy, stylish ski parka go from the outrageous price of $300 to the astronomical price of $500 in a matter of seven months. Other parkas that provided more warmth were considerably cheaper and much more appropriate for children. The difference was that the cheaper parka didn't have a "French cut" and wasn't manufactured by an "in" ski clothes company. Shop around for the best values. Good ski clothes for children should be warm, but not too bulky. Ski swaps (places where you can buy and exchange used clothing and equipment) are great places to get clothes at reasonable prices—let somebody else pay the markup.

Boots are the most important equipment you can buy for your child for skiing or snowboarding. Boots should be warm, provide good support, and above all, fit well. Try to get boots that are easy to put on and take off. An ill-fitting pair will hamper learning and may cause injury. Inquire at various ski shops about children's equipment trade-ins. You may be able to get your child new boots every season at a reasonable price.

Bindings are also very important. Be sure to use children's because they are adjusted for skiers with lower body weight. Adult bindings may not release for a 50-pound skier. If you buy used bindings at a swap, be sure they're lubricated and work properly.

Skis and snowboards should be appropriate for the age and ability level of the child. They should be flexible and short enough so the child can maneuver with them. A ski shop with a good children's department can help you choose an appropriate pair of skies.

• Make sure your child is adequately supervised on the hill. Children shouldn't be allowed to venture off by themselves until they have had some experience. Mountains can be very unforgiving places: snow storms or even cold winds can cause frostbite or hypothermia (low body temperature), and obstacles such as trees or lift towers can cause injuries to the unwary young skier.

Many ski areas have nursery or youth ski programs that provide babysitting and ski lessons at the same time. A whole day of this service can be expensive, so use it when you want to get in some concentrated skiing, and then enjoy teaching and skiing with your children.

• Make sure your children are comfortable. They should wear sunscreens, sunglasses, and appropriate clothing. Be sure their equipment is operating correctly. Boots that won't buckle or bindings that won't work can be frustrating and dangerous to a child and can ruin an otherwise exciting experience. Remember that children can fatigue suddenly. They also get cold more quickly than adults. Take a break from time to time. A hot chocolate or a glass of juice can provide a brief respite from skiing or snowboarding and will help the kids last a lot longer.

- Children like to learn by example. Don't over-intellectualize about skiing or snowboarding technique. Ski down the hill and encourage them to imitate you. Have patience—even Olympic skiers were beginners at one time.

Cross-Country Skiing

Cross-country skiing can serve as an excellent introduction to winter sports for children and families. Where the expense of downhill skiing can be prohibitive, cross-country skiing can be learned relatively inexpensively. It's easy to involve small children in a family cross-country skiing outing. When a child gets tired, he or she can be carried in a backpack.

It's best to rent equipment the first few times. This will give you the opportunity to learn which equipment is best for you and your family.

Start with relatively short trips on flat terrain. Children should begin learning to walk with the skis on—you can get a head start by practicing at home. You may want to go to cross-country ski parks the first few times; they often have manicured ski trails that greatly facilitate learning. As learning progresses, introduce skiing up and down hills. As with any winter sport, try to maximize your child's comfort. And remember that children fatigue easily; if you push a child too hard, you can turn a potentially positive experience into a nightmare.

Sledding, Tubing, Tobogganing

Although these activities are traditional favorites with children, they can be potentially dangerous if you don't take proper precautions. Many parents who shudder at the thought of their children skiing think nothing of letting them careen down a local hill. The neighborhood sled run may have unforeseen hazards, whereas ski runs are usually manicured to the point of being very safe.

Make sure your kids check a hill before venturing down it with a sled. Bumps that cause a child to become airborne can result in spinal injury.

Ice Skating

Ice skating is a great family activity that, because of indoor rinks, can be practiced year-round in even the warmest climates. The best way to begin is to include children in ice skating parties with family and friends. It's probably easiest for children to learn with figure skates because they provide more ankle support than speed skates or hockey skates do. If the child shows further interest, then he or she can take lessons in more advanced techniques. Ice skating can be used for conditioning if the child has room for continuous, vigorous movement.

Camping and Backpacking

These activities are very enjoyable lifetime sports. After an initial investment in equipment, families have an activity at their disposal that will provide not only enjoyment, but also a vehicle for physical fitness and togetherness. As with other family activities, begin with short, simple outings. Start by camping in areas you can drive to. Most states have camping grounds with the conveniences of home. As children learn basic camping skills, then the family is ready for more challenging backpacking trips.

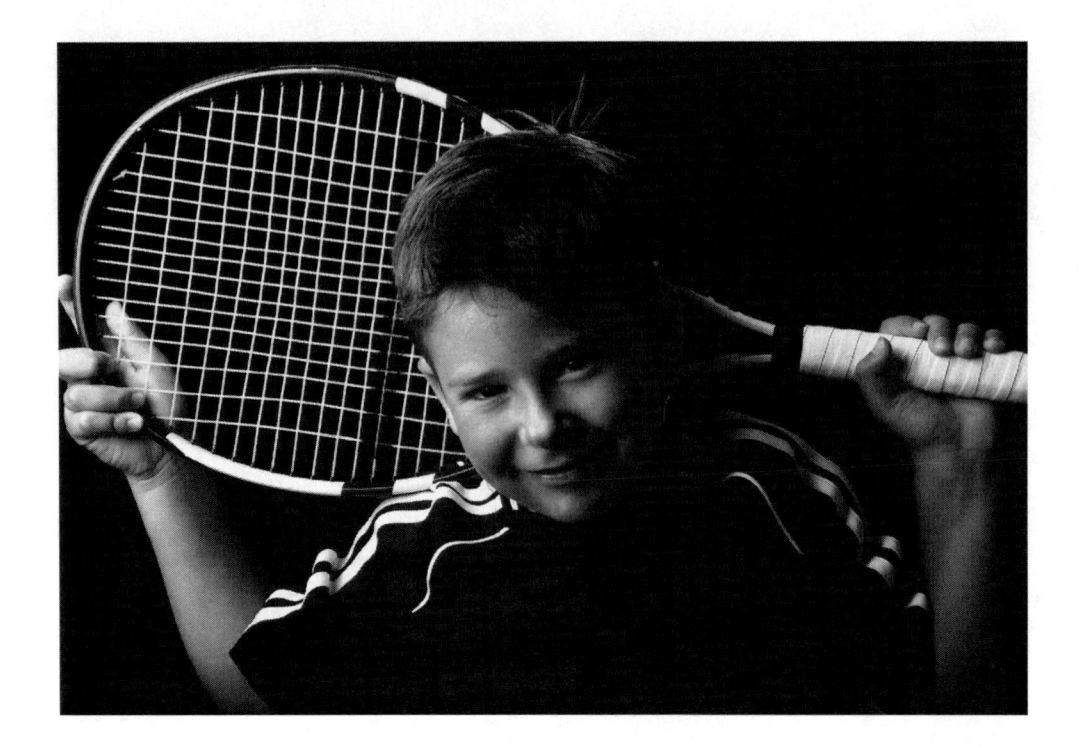

Equipment is very important in backpacking. In fact, it's better to rent good equipment than to purchase some that's inferior in quality. Poor quality equipment can cause a lot of discomfort, and usually falls apart. A backpack with poorly designed straps can dig into a child's shoulders, making him miserable. The most important items for a young camper are sleeping bag and boots. Boots should have a slip-resistant sole. Sleeping bags should provide adequate warmth. New synthetic materials are available that provide almost as much warmth as the more expensive down sleeping bags. The money you spend on a bag really depends on the kind of camping you're contemplating—winter camping requires a much better bag than you'll need for camping during the summer. A good pack that fits well is also very desirable. If your child is very young, it's probably better if you carry some of his equipment. Let him carry a light "day pack" so that he can experience the satisfaction of participation.

As with other lifetime sports, always try to make the experience positive. Start off with short hikes from a central base camp. As the child gains experience, the backpacking trips can become longer. Take frequent rest stops, and be sure your child gets plenty of water and nourishment.

Recreational Ball Sports

These are probably the most popular sports in the United States. Taken as a group, sports like tennis, golf, racquetball, basketball, softball, and volleyball account for the largest percentage of the recreational dollar. I've already discussed school sports such as basketball and softball, so I'll concentrate here on activities traditionally learned outside school.

Tennis

Although you can teach your child to play tennis, he or she will make the fastest progress by learning from a professional instructor who specializes in teaching children. Tennis is a difficult sport to learn, and children younger than eight or nine lack the basic coordination and strength required for it. Before this age, it's better to work on basic ball-handling skills (see Chapter 2).

Good tennis teachers involve children in enjoyable games that teach the fundamentals almost by accident. Bouncing the ball against the racquet and tennis relay races serve to develop racquet and ball-handling skills without pressuring children to progress to difficult forehand or backhand shots. As children develop dexterity with the racquet, skills are learned more easily.

As in other sports, equipment is important. Racquets should be appropriate to the body weight and strength of the child. An ill-fitting racquet will make learning difficult and injuries almost inevitable. Tennis can be modified for the young novice; techniques such as lowering the net can do much to develop skills and confidence.

Racquetball, Handball, Squash

These sports require a great deal of coordination and a high level of fitness. For these reasons, children shouldn't begin learning them until they're eight or nine years old. These sports can serve as good learning activities for tennis—because the games are played in an enclosed space, the ball has fewer places to go and so it is easier to hit.

Volleyball

This is a great sport for family outings and picnics. Volleyball can be used to develop ball-handling skills in children. Children can begin learning this sport by tossing the ball up in the air and catching it. Then they can progress to a low net—throwing the ball to one another over it. As your child becomes better at handling the ball, he or she can begin to work on specific volleyball skills.

Golf

Children can learn golf at about eight years old. I would strongly urge you to take your child to a driving range before going out on a golf course. Some lessons from a golf pro can do much to develop basic fundamentals in children. With practice on the driving range and lessons from a pro, your child can venture out on a course and have fun without being a nuisance to adults.

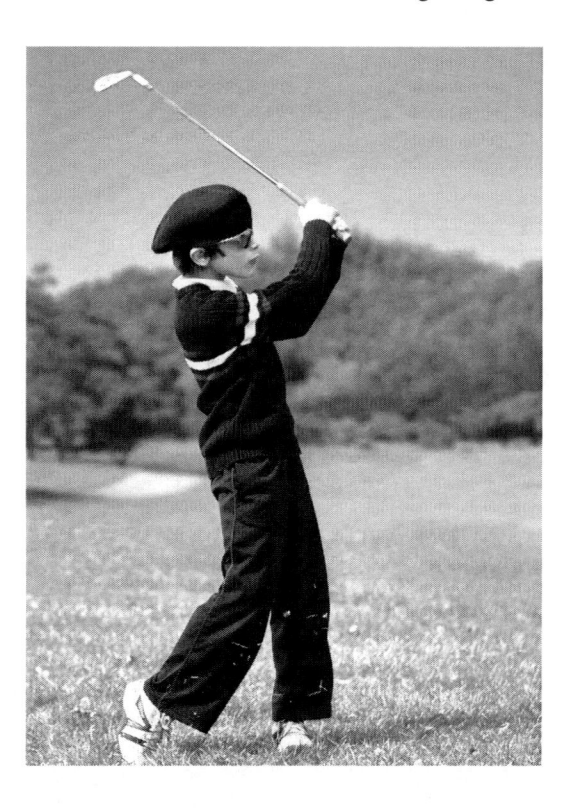

DEVELOPING AN ACTIVE LIFESTYLE

A nine hole "chip-and-putt" course is probably the best to begin on. These courses often have special rates for kids, especially at midweek. Because they cater to the less skilled, chip-and-putt courses are usually more conducive to your child's early effort.

"Pee-wee golf"—putting around obstacles—can provide family recreation and develop golf skills at the same time. Although pee-wee golf courses are found principally in resort communities, many residential areas, particularly in the suburbs, have them as well.

A golf tournament is the most common type of business athletic event (although running races are certainly becoming more popular). Golf skills can definitely be a social asset.

New Sports

The sports we play have changed in the past 20 years. While many young people skied, now most want to snowboard. Sports like in-line skating, rock climbing on climbing walls, step aerobics, lacrosse, and ultimate frisbee—that barely existed until recently—have legions of avid participants. The most important thing is to find sports and physical activities that you and your child enjoy and do them.

Putting Sports in Perspective

Sports and physical activity are important for children whether they participate in organized athletics or not. Physical activity is necessary for the development of healthy bodies and emotional and psychological growth. If children learn the skills for a few lifetime sports, they'll carry their learning and love of playing into adulthood. Sports and physical activity can become habits for a lifetime if the experiences children have when they're young are good ones. Help your children learn to love being active. They'll be happier, healthier kids, and they'll thank you for it when they are trim, fit, fun-loving adults!

Instant Replay

- Lifetime sports, physical activities carried over from childhood to adulthood, should be stressed for the athlete and the non-athlete alike.

- Lifetime exercise habits should be developed during childhood. Lifetime exercise programs should include development of endurance, strength, flexibility, and skill.

- Suggested lifetime sports include running, swimming, tennis, golf, skiing, racquetball, backpacking, and scuba diving Just to name a few).

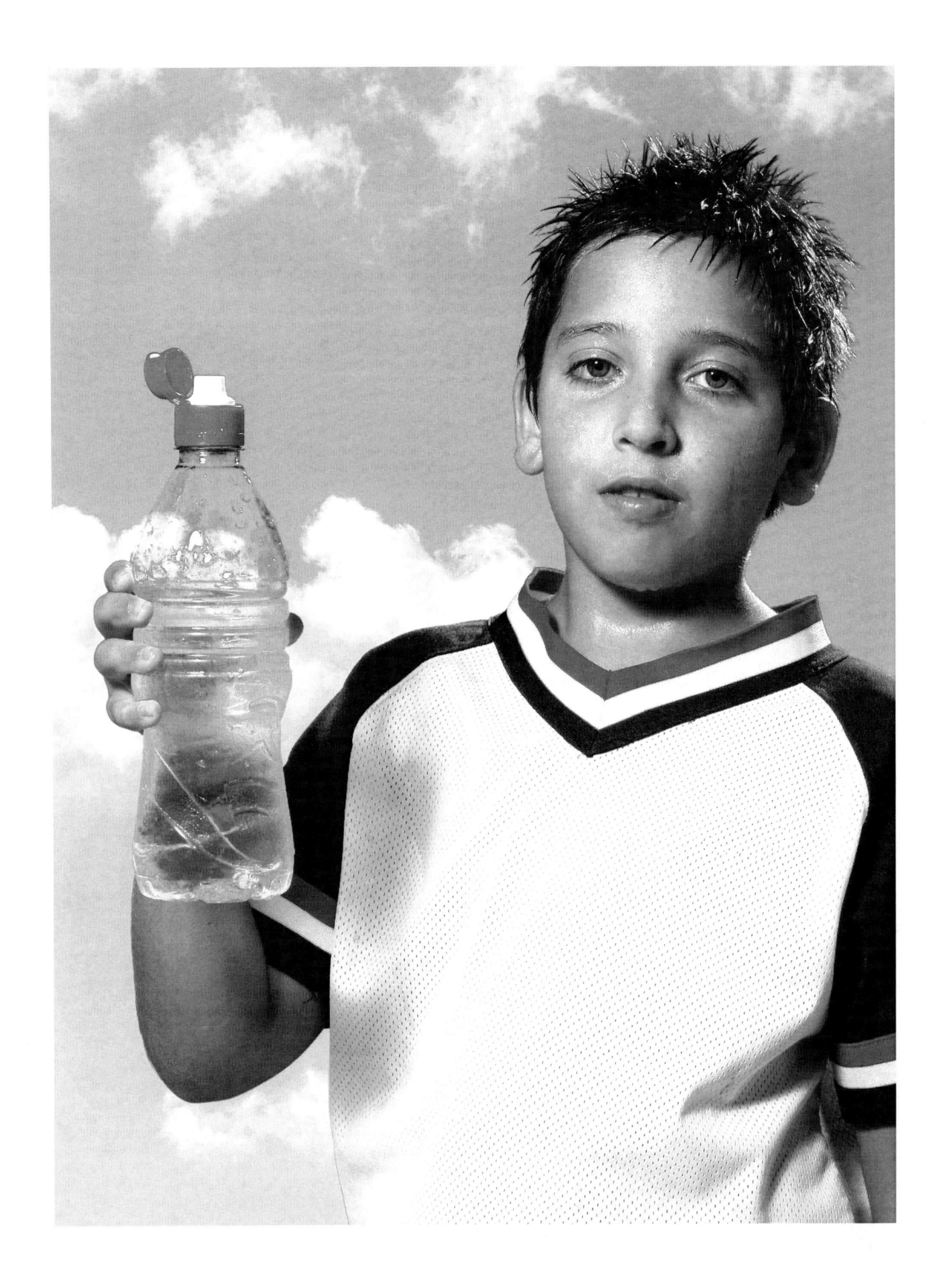

Index

Achilles tendon stretch, 77
Adolescence, 59-87
    determining target heart rate in, 65-66, 87
    developing endurance in, 64-70, 87
    developing flexibility in, 74-77, 87
    developing speed and agility in, 71-74
    developing strength in, 78-87
    interval training in, 71-73, 87
    measuring maximal heart rate in, 65-66
    motor development in, 62-64
    running program in, 69-70
    short-term running goals in, 67-68
    social factors in, 62
    sports ability in, 63
    well-rounded physical fitness in, 64
Agility, 71
Agility exercise, 73
Amphetamines, 98
Anabolic steroids, 98, 101-104
Asthma, 122-123
Astrand, Per-Olaf, 21
Athletics, competitive, 89-107
    East German myth and, 102
    emotional elements in, 99
    girls and, 106-107
    involvement in, 96-99
    maximizing child's experience in, 99-102
    nutrition and, 105
    physical aspects of, 11, 99
    proper perspective on, 101-102, 107
    science and, 102-105, 107
    selecting sports for, 90-96, 107
    training and, 100-101
    see also specific sports

Backpacking, 133-134
Back rolls, 75
Balance skills, 27-31, 44, 47-49
Ball-handling skills, 53-54
Ball sports, recreational, 134-136
Bench press, 84
Bent-knee sit-ups, 79
Biceps curls, 85
Bicycling, 47-48
Bill of Rights for Young Athletes, 107
Blood pressure, 62
Blood supplementation (blood doping), 103
Boating, 130
Body fat, control of, 20, 126-127
Body image, 28, 44, 51

Camping, 133-134
Camps, sports, 101-102
Cardiovascular fitness, 19-20, 31, 47, 64, 67
Catching, 45, 53-54, 57
Childhood, 32-57
    balance and proprioception in, 47-49
    coordination in, 39, 43-45, 49-50, 54-55
    developing basic skills in, 56
    different growth rates in, 34-35
    motor development in, 41-54
    movement experiences in, 34, 56, 57
    movement and sports exercises in, 46
    skill refinement in, 45-46
Chin-ups (pull-ups), 80
Climbing, 43-44, 49, 52
Coaches, dealing with, 98-99
Coaching, injury prevention and, 109-111, 123
Competition, 14-16, 18, 19, 31, 94-98, 107

Coordination, 23, 28-31, 49-52
Creeping and crawling skills, 41
Cryokinetics, 116
Cybex, 26
Cycling skills, 47-48

Directionality, 28
Diving, 129

Elementary-school physical education program, 55-56, 57
Endurance fitness, 18-22, 31
Epiphyseal plates (growth plates), 35
    injuries to, 36, 120-121, 123
Equipment and playing surfaces, advances in, 103
Ergogenic aids, 103-105
Exercise heart rate, 66-67
Exercise machines, 103

Family environment, 16
Family participation, 19, 31
Fitness-oriented sports, 91, 92
Flexibility, 26, 31, 64, 74-77, 87, 127
Foot/eye coordination, 29, 55
Footsies, 77

Galloping, 43
Glycogen, 119
Golf, 135-136
Groin stretches, 75
Growth plate injuries, 36, 120-121, 123
Gymnasiums:
    home, 81-82, 87
    public, 82, 87
    school, 86-87
Gymnastics, 48-49, 56

Hand/eye coordination, 28, 29, 31, 37, 38, 45, 50, 54, 55
Handball, 135
Health clubs, 82, 87
Heart disease, 18, 19, 20, 22, 31, 62, 64, 86
Heart rate, exercise, 66-67, 87
Heart rate, maximal, 65
    measuring of, 65
    target heart rate determined from, 66
Heart rate, target, 65, 87
    use of, 66-67
Heel raises, 79
High school physical education program, 86-87
Hip stretches, 76
Home gymnasium:
    components of, 81-82
    safety in, 82, 87
Hopping, 43
Hormones, muscle fitness and, 23-24
Hurdler stretch, 76
Hyperplasia, 35
Hypertrophy, 35

Ice skating, 133
Imbalance injuries, 119-120, 123
Infancy, 33-41
    motor development in, 37-41, 57
    movement exercises in, 38-41
    perceptual development in, 37-39, 57
Injuries and disabilities, 109-123
    common in children's sports, 116-122
    consulting physician for, 115
    good equipment and, 113-123
    growth plate and, 120-121, 123
    from imbalance, 119-120, 123
    to joints and muscles, 116-118
    medical supervision and, 113-115
    from overuse, 118-119, 123

parents and, 111-113
prevention of, 109-115
proper coaching and, 109-111, 123
rehabilitation of, 117-118
treatment of, 116-117
Interval training, 71

Jumpers, 40
Jumping, 43
Jumping rope, 49

Kindergyms, 40
Kinesthesis, 28
Knee bends, 79

Laterality, 28
Leg exercises, 78-79
Lifetime sports, 133, 134, 136

Maximal oxygen consumption test, 20-21
Mononucleosis, 121-122
Movement experiences, 12, 27, 28, 29, 31, 33, 37, 38, 40, 43, 44, 49, 56
Movement-oriented sports, 91
Movement skills, 14, 22, 27, 28, 29, 30, 31, 33, 34, 36, 37, 38, 41, 43, 45, 46, 47, 51, 55, 56
Muscle fibers, 23
Muscle fitness, role of hormones in, 23-24
Muscle strength, 22-24, 31, 127

Nutrition, 105

Ogilvie, Bruce, 12
Olympic development training centers, 22
Osgood-Schlatter disease, 121
Oxygen, breathing of, 105

Parachute, exercise with, 50-51
Parallel bar dips, 80
Perceptual-motor skills, 27-31, 55
Phantom chair exercise, 78
Physical education programs:
    in elementary school, 55-56, 57
    in high school, 86-87
Power, exercise training and, 22-24
Proprioception, 38, 40, 45, 47-49
Protein supplements, 104
Puberty, 13, 19, 22, 24, 34, 35, 46, 57, 59-62, 78, 81, 95
    body changes in, 60-62
    see also Adolescence
Pullovers, 85
Push-ups, 80, 81

Racquetball, 134, 135, 136
Recruitment, muscle fiber, 23
River rafting, 130
Roller-skating, 48
Running:
    heart rate and, 65
    interval training in, 71-73
    program for, 69-70
    short-term goals in, 67-68
    skills in, 36, 43, 47, 54, 55

Safety:
    of athletics, 96
    in balancing activities, 47-49
    in home gymnasium, 82
    in water activities, 128, 130
    in winter sports, 132
    see also Injuries and disabilities
Scuba diving, 129-130, 136
Self-image, positive, 55-56
Shin stretches, 77

Shoulder circles with a towel, 77
Shoulder hangs, 76
Side bends, 80
Sitting stretches, 74
Skateboarding, 44, 48
Skiing:
    cross-country, 133
    snow, 44, 131-133
    water, 44, 130
Skipping, 43
Sledding, 131, 133
Speed, 22-24, 31, 71, 87
Speed exercises, 73-74
Sports camps, 101-102
Sports clubs, selection of, 96-98
Squash, 135
Squats, 83, 84
Stair climbing, 79
Step-ups, 79
Stomach exercises, 79-80
Strength training, 78-86, 87
   without equipment, 78-80
   with weights, 81-86
Surfing, 129
Swimming, 125, 128-129, 136

Technique-oriented sports, 91, 93
Tennis, 134, 135
Testosterone, 23-24
Throwing, 14, 41, 43, 45, 53-54, 57
Tobogganing, 131, 133
Trampolines, 48
Treadmill tests, 18, 21-22
Tubing, 133
Twists, 80

Upper body exercises, 80

Visual ability, 29
Visual-motor control, 29
Vitamin supplements, 104
Volleyball, 134, 135

Walking, 37, 41, 43, 46-47, 49
Water skiing, 130
Water sports, 128-131
Weight problems, 20, 63, 127
Weight training, 22, 24-26, 61, 81-83, 86
   basic exercises in, 83-86
   equipment, 81-82
   principles of, 82-83
What to do about athletic injuries, 111-115
Winning, 13-16
Winter sports, 131-133
Wrist curls, 85